THE ROAD I NEVER MEANT TO TAKE

REAL STORIES. REAL SCIENCE. REAL RECOVERY.

"I got sober because I wanted a better life. I stay sober because I got one."

BY ALANNA BELL

The Road I Never Meant to Take: Real Stories. Real Science. Real Recovery.
Published by SWI Publishing
Broomfield, CO

ISBN: 979-8-9996331-1-8 (paperback)
        979-8-9996331-2-5 (hardback)
        979-8-9996331-0-1 (ebook)

BIOGRAPHY & AUTOBIOGRAPHY / Social Scientists & Psychologists
SELF-HELP / Substance Abuse & Addictions / Alcohol

Cover design by Alanna Bell. Copyright owned by Alanna Bell.

This book is based on the author's personal experiences and the experiences of those she has worked with in a therapeutic setting. To protect privacy, certain names, identifying details, and circumstances have been changed.

QUANTITY PURCHASES: Schools, companies, professional groups, clubs, and other organizations may qualify for special terms when ordering quantities of this title. For information, email info@AlannaBellWrites.com.

Printed in the United States of America.

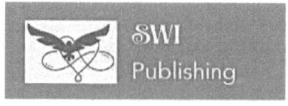

Praises for The Road I Never Meant to Take

"The Road I Never Meant to Take is a powerful and emotionally moving read. The author skillfully weaves a personal story of addiction and mental health struggles with compassion and honesty. I especially appreciated the thoughtful inclusion of scientific insights and modern treatment approaches, which added depth and relevance to the narrative. This book offers a strong message of hope—for recovery from addiction and mental health challenges, as well as for coping with grief and loss."

— **Dr. Chuck Smith**
Author of Understanding Addiction: Know Science, No Stigma.
Addiction Medicine Specialist | Speaker | Recovery Advocate

"This book is a standout in recovery literature. Its story has been lived by many but has not been held up to the light, and shared. Alanna has done this with candor, bravery, kindness, and deep clinical understanding. The second-person address is intimate and heart-wrenching, and models the self-reflection and vulnerability required for healing. Alanna gives us all of it, with unflinching clarity and kindness."

— **Kate Small, BA, MS** Special Education Teacher

"When your life becomes your laboratory, every day offers new lessons. I've always loved learning from the ordinary moments in my own life—and Alanna does this beautifully. In The Road I Never Meant to Take, she shares her hard-earned insights with honesty and heart, inspiring us to discover the lessons in our own stories."

— **Michael Malone, MA, MFT, ACHt** Therapist, Coach, Teacher

"The Road I Never Meant to Take is a profound bridge between the science of healing and the soul of recovery. As someone trained in neuroscience and deeply committed to mind-body wellness, I found Alanna's integration of trauma,

addiction science, and spirituality to be both accurate and powerfully human. But beyond the science, this book made me feel. It reminded me why I do the work I do—and why so many healers are quietly suffering. Alanna's letters are not just for readers in recovery; they're for anyone who has ever lost themselves while trying to save others."

— Ashlie Bell, PhD, LCSW, QEEG-DL, BCN
Founder of NeuroGrove Integrative Brain Wellness Center

"The Road I Never Meant to Take is a powerful and thought-provoking read. It expanded my understanding of substance use disorder and led me to reflect deeply on my own life, my loved ones, and the choices we make along the way."

— John Horat, PE
Owner/CEO, Bitterroot Engineering and Design

"For anyone whose life has been touched by substance use disorder (and really, that's all of us), this book is a treasure trove of poetic wisdom, heartfelt stories, and powerful truths. Through deeply personal reflections and evidence-based insights, the author— herself a therapist in recovery—shares, through the character known only as 'L', how she transformed a life of pain and anger into one filled with joy and purpose. Read it slowly, like a meditation, and let it illuminate the wisdom already within you."

— Teresa Bou-Matar, LPC
Licensed Professional Counselor, School Counselor (Retired)

"This book is beautifully written. With each chapter, you feel like you're a part of the story—experiencing what the author is feeling. From fighting back tears and laughing out loud to feeling anxious about what happens next, you're offered a clear, visceral glimpse of what it means to truly live."

— TSgt Stacie J. Hyche, USAF (Retired Medic), RT(S), RDMS
Sonographer/Ultrasound Technician

Dedication

To my family—
for your love, your laughter, and your presence through it all.
And to the silent sufferers—
this book is for you.

May these pages be a rope in the dark,
a quiet voice that says:
You're not alone. There is another way. Hope lives.

Author's Note

I never meant to write a book.

I meant to survive.

In the early days of my recovery, I started writing letters—quiet, unfiltered reflections I never intended to share. They were written from the heart of my healing process, when I was still unraveling shame, still learning to stay. These letters helped me find my footing. They helped me stay sober. They helped me begin again.

Over time, the voice of these letters took on a shape of her own.

I called her **L**.

L is not me, and yet she is made of pieces of me—of clients I've walked beside, colleagues I've mourned, and every brave soul who has dared to heal while still holding space for others. L is the therapist who should have known better. The professional who kept showing up. The human who finally broke open.

These letters are not instructions—but you may find guidance or direction within them.

They are not formulas— but important research and scientific truths are here to deepen your understanding.

They are not always pretty—but if you look closely, you may find beauty in the process of becoming whole.

These pages are not polished. They're honest.

And they are offered with the hope that they will meet you where you are—whether you are in recovery, love someone who is, or are simply searching for your own way home.

Healing takes time.

It twists. It speaks. It moves in unexpected ways.

It's not always quiet.

But it is always possible.

And telling the truth—even in fragments—can save a life.

Thank you for letting me share my healing journey.

May these letters help you discover the shape of your own.

— **Alanna Bell**

Table of Contents

Introduction

Get ready for a different kind of recovery story. One told not through dry statistics or clinical advice, but through raw, tender, and sometimes laugh-out-loud letters from a therapist who has walked both sides of the healing path.

This is a book to be taken in slowly and savored. Though the stories read like a memoir, each letter stands on its own—an adventure in insight, a truth offered in vulnerability, a moment meant for reflection.

These 52 letters were written with intention—not just to tell my story, but to invite you into your own. They come from the inside—from the trenches of substance use disorder, the winding road of recovery, and the quiet beauty of becoming whole again. Some are fiery. Some are soft. All are honest. All are meant to be digested one at a time.

Consider reading one per day—or one per week. Let each letter breathe. Reflect. Journal. Share them with a friend or colleague. Let your own questions rise.

Whether you're a professional in the helping fields, someone in recovery, or someone trying to understand a loved one's struggle, these letters are for you. You'll find stories that speak to the mind, the body, and the soul. You'll also find evidence-based insights woven throughout—science made personal, psychology made human, spirituality grounded in real life.

These letters are more than just a chronicle of one person's journey. They're a companion for anyone walking a path toward greater wholeness. My hope is that, somewhere between the pages, you'll find your own breath catching, your heart softening, and your perspective shifting.

Recovery isn't just about stopping something. It's about becoming someone.

And healing—real healing—takes time.

So take your time.

Let the road rise to meet you.

And remember—you don't have to walk it alone.

- *L*

1. Joy Ride

Wow. What a beautiful morning in Colorado. I had so much fun driving my new bright blue jeep through the mountains with the top down, the wind tangling my hair in that glorious "I should've tied it up" kind of way. The air smelled of pine and warm earth, and I had to slow down more than once for deer and elk lingering at the roadside, who were watching me like they were considering hitching a ride. The warm shower of sunshine flowed down onto my head and shoulders, with just enough clouds to keep it from burning my skin. And there were so many birds! They were everywhere. From the hawks soaring through the air to the smaller flocks flitting between the trees, all seemed to be on their way to join a big avian block party.

I recreated our favorite travel playlist before I left–you know, just in case reception cut out (which, of course, it did). But nothing was going to dampen my joy today. I just turned up the music, sang along at the top of my lungs, and let myself feel completely, fully alive.

I wish you'd been here to enjoy it with me. I know you would have loved it. You always loved the open road and that feeling of escape it gave to us. I smiled as I replayed the fun and laughter of our many expeditions. And yet, as I was driving, another ride also kept pushing its way into my mind.

The last time I took this road—over two years ago—I wasn't the one driving. My sister was. I was in the passenger seat, shaking, drowning in shame, barely holding myself together. The nausea was unbearable, though it had nothing to do with the winding roads. The truth is, I barely remember the scenery that day. I only remember the weight of my despair.

You know as well as anyone what that kind of despair feels like. As therapists, we spend so much time trying to help others, but when we're struggling ourselves, it's easy to feel like we're failing—not just as people, but in our profession. That day, I felt like I'd hit rock bottom, both personally and professionally.

You understand what I mean when I say *dark*, and that drive was darker than anything I had ever known.

I had actually finished off a bottle of wine first thing that morning—not for fun, not for a buzz, but rather to numb myself enough to keep from backing out of going into rehab. To keep myself from screaming or sobbing or losing my mind altogether. To quiet the voices of shame taunting me in my head.

Truth is, every day was rough back then. I think back on a typical day, when the worst season of my addiction had me in a chokehold with barely enough air to breathe. I'd wake up around 4 a.m. with nausea and the shakes, my body demanding a drink before I could do anything else. I didn't even pretend anymore. I would gulp straight from the bottle, knowing it was the only way I'd be able to settle down enough to go back to sleep. Depending on my schedule, I would either force myself into the shower, pulling myself together to perform my functional duties for work or family—or I would just give up entirely and drink from dawn to dark.

While the rest of the house was still asleep, I'd look in the mirror with disgust. I would stare at the tired bloodshot eyes, the puffy face, the lifeless skin, the shell of the person I once was. I was sick in my body. Sick in my mind. Sick in my heart.

Sure, I could function sometimes—if I had to. I could show up to work, smile at my family, hold a conversation without slurring my words. But underneath it all, I was rotting. I was depressed, frustrated, and so ashamed of who I had become.

By the time my sister drove me to rehab, I was so depressed I didn't even know if I wanted to keep living. I'd tried to quit drinking so many times on my own, with doctors, therapists, even friends like you cheering me on. But nothing worked for longer than a week or two. I didn't want to admit I needed more help. As a therapist, that seemed like the ultimate failure.

When I finally surrendered and walked into Harmony Recovery Center, I was convinced it was my last shot. I honestly can't remember if you'd ever mentioned that place back when we were seeking referrals for our clients, but the folks there literally saved my life. Walking in with my head down, refusing eye contact in my shame, I had expected judgment, condescension, maybe even pity. Instead, they offered only kindness with a genuine desire to help me.

I had spoken with one of the admissions counselors several times on the phone before finally going in, and he made sure he was there to greet me during my admission. Even when the staff had to give me the breathalyzer and go through my belongings, somehow, they normalized it. I felt humiliated, but they took away some of the sting. Regardless of what I might have seen when I looked in the mirror, they seemed to see something better. They somehow made me feel *almost* respectable—something I hadn't felt in a long time.

Then came detox. That part terrified me. But the nurses were like angels in scrubs. They didn't pity me or scold me; they just treated me like a human being who deserved care. The doctors were lighthearted but professional, and they made sure I was comfortable, giving me the appropriate medications to help me through the detoxification process. After a quick tour, they tucked me into a bed where I slept for what felt like a week, though it was only a day or two.

The rest of the rehab property was made up of a lovely set of cabins with a couple of central group rooms and hang out spaces. There was a separate large dining hall that doubled as an auditorium for large meetings, trainings, and celebrations. The program was so well run that, while it was difficult admitting to and working through the pains of addiction, it was also, in a strange way, like a retreat. It was an opportunity to escape all the other pressures and expectations in my life—for a whole month—and just work on me. Talk about a first!

When I walked in that door, I honestly didn't believe I could ever return to the level of peace I feel today. In fact, I'm not sure I ever even felt joy like this in my life before the addiction took hold. You know all the years I suffered, having no idea if things would ever be better, but moving through the steps to get sober brought me to this new and wondrous place of being.

I wish you were here to take this joyride with me. We've always had the best adventures together. I know you've had your own battles with alcohol, so you know the suffering it can bring. What a contrast to the bliss I feel today. You always said you wanted to feel alive again. I think about that a lot—about how we both dreamed of better days, even when we didn't believe they were possible.

15

Looking down at my keychain, I read the words aloud. It says, "I got sober because I wanted a better life. I stay sober because I got one." When I bought this, I only hoped it would be true. I can't say that I expected it. Yet here I am. The only thing that would have made this day better would be having you here with me. We've always had so much fun together. For now, just imagine my smile and I'll imagine yours! I miss you!

Sending my love...

- *L*

2. Girl's Night

Last night was magical. Four generations—my granddaughters, my daughter, my mom, and me—laughing, playing, making memories together. We had sushi, watched movies, and let silliness fill the air. Even at 87, my mom could be as playful as the girls, giggling right alongside them. I soaked it in, holding onto each moment. I wish you could have been here, you would've fit right in. You always had a knack for making people laugh.

It's incredible to think about how much has changed. Not so long ago, my drinking cost me opportunities like this. Once my family realized I had a serious problem, they stopped trusting me to care for my mom or my granddaughters. At the time, I was furious, but deep down, I knew they were right.

Even though I told myself I wasn't drunk or wasted, I was often "off" enough to be a risk. I might not have been safe to drive in an emergency or make critical decisions if something went wrong. Looking back, I see how much I minimized the impact of my drinking—convincing myself I was still responsible, even when my judgment was clearly compromised. You know the mental gymnastics we can pull off to protect our illusions of control.

I couldn't see it then, but I can now: they weren't punishing me. They were protecting themselves and their loved ones. It's such a painful reality to face—those boundaries that feel like walls. You know exactly what I mean. I remember how devastated you were when your family cut you off after your sister's wedding. I remember your pain, your shame—because I felt it, too. The deep, gut-wrenching knowledge that your actions had made people afraid to trust you.

It's hard to describe that kind of heartbreak to someone who hasn't lived it. I have always loved my family so much, and if ever there was a reason to get sober, you'd think this would be it. You'd think love would be enough. But we both know addiction doesn't work that way.

How many times did we swear we would stop? How many times did we grit our teeth, make the vow, tell ourselves we'd just use willpower—only to fail, again and again? I spent years thinking it was just me. That I was weak. That I lacked self-control. That I was, ultimately, a failure.

Then, in rehab, I read the book *Under the Influence*, and for the first time, I understood what was happening to me. I learned that, for some of us(more than ten percent of the population, across ethnic and socio-economic lines), our bodies react to alcohol in an entirely abnormal way. It's not just about bad choices or a lack of willpower. It's biological.

Let me tell you what happens:

- When alcohol enters our system, it disrupts normal biochemical processes, throwing off our enzymes, hormones, and neurotransmitters.
- Our mitochondria—our cells' powerhouses—start changing to adapt to the alcohol. They become so efficient at using alcohol as fuel that they prefer it over actual food.
- Over time, our cells—now dependent on alcohol—begin to deteriorate. The delicate chemical balance is destroyed. The membranes break down. The entire system starts to collapse from the inside out.

What blew my mind most was realizing this isn't a matter of willpower. The cellular changes start immediately, not after years of abuse like I'd been led to believe. I was always under the impression that a person became an alcoholic because they drank too much, for too long, and that it was the repeated drinking that changed their body. But that isn't what scientific evidence shows!

I can't help but wonder, why did I have to go to rehab to learn this? Why isn't this front and center in the medical and mental health fields? Why isn't this common knowledge? What if I had known this earlier? What if I had understood, before it was too late, that my brain and body were set up differently? That my drinking wasn't just a bad habit, but a disease hijacking my cells and brain pathways?

In any case, here's the thing: now that I know better, I'm doing better. Nights like last night are proof of that. And after the movies, we continued our delightful fun into the morning. We all made waffles together, topping them with berries and whipped cream. I've never seen so many giggles over sticky fingers and overflowing batter.

This morning, as I sit here in the quiet house, the girls back at their home and my mom resting peacefully in her room, I can't stop smiling at the waffle batter still on the counter and the dishes piled up in the sink. Life feels so full these days.

You know, my mom receives in-home hospice care now, so time with her feels especially precious. I don't take any of it for granted—every hug, every laugh, every shared meal. And if I hadn't gotten sober, I would have missed these precious moments—the way she threw her head back in laughter, the way she reached across the table to sneak an extra bite of whipped cream.

And the girls are growing up so fast. I'm so grateful I didn't miss out on these moments. The laughter, the messiness, the pure joy—these are the things worth fighting for.

I don't take it for granted. Not one bit. I could have missed out on this life entirely. But as it turns out, life today is actually quite wonderful.. The only thing that would have made it even better is if you had been here to join us! For now, feel the love and giggles I am sending your way.

- *L*

3. Badge of Honor

You'll never believe what we've been up to this week! By "we," I mean all three grandkids and myself. We're just about to wrap up a *birthday week extravaganza*. Two of the kids turned 13, one hit double digits, and—well, let's just say my birthday was in the mix, too. (No need to dwell on that particular number!) We went all out with big adventure plans, and we weren't disappointed.

We started at Six Flags, where we braved the scariest roller coaster rides. Then there were sleepovers every night at our house, full of games, movies, and zooming around our neighborhood park on electric scooters. And just when we thought we couldn't pack in more fun, we hit Waterworld, where we took on some of the biggest water slides in the country.

I have to tell you—I'm pretty sure I was the oldest lady out there doing the rides. You'd have cracked up watching me literally need to *roll* out of a group raft after everyone else gracefully stepped out of it. But you know what? I actually take pride in being "that lady." It's a badge of honor!

It's funny, though. Being the oldest on the waterslides felt very different from being the oldest in rehab—not to mention the only one from the mental health field. I remember being puzzled by this at first, but then it hit me: by the time someone reaches my age, they've often given up or given in to the condition. Either they resign themselves to a slow decline, or the disease takes them quickly in one way or another. Truth is, if someone suffers with a substance use disorder starting from a younger age, and they don't get help, they usually don't live to be as old as I am.

And then there's the shame. You and I have talked about how stigma and misinformation run deep, especially in our field. For centuries, and unfortunately still, there is a common belief that addiction is mostly a psychological disorder. Most therapists don't end up in public rehab. Instead, they quit their careers—or worse. You know exactly what I mean.

And I get it. I was terrified before confessing I needed help and resigning myself to getting it. I knew there was a real chance I could lose my license and career. Counseling has been my calling and my passion. I spent years of blood, sweat, and tears pouring into this career, not to mention the huge financial investment of earning my master's degree, all while working full time and raising a family. Facing the possibility of losing it all was gut wrenching. It felt unbearable.

Did I tell you about the time I even reached out to the state mental health board? I was desperate to see if they had any kind of support or guidance for a struggling provider like me. They didn't. Oh, they have the rules, the protocols, the guidelines for reporting, even assessments and evaluations to determine whether you're fit to practice after you get treatment—but no actual *support*. Nothing to help you get to the point of being sober and healthy enough to face those evaluations. It felt so cold, like they were only waiting for me to fail so they could revoke my license.

And yet, living the lie of being "well" when I was falling apart was worse. I couldn't keep up the facade anymore. You know all the books we've read, training we've had on shame and the cycles of addiction, but none of it prepared me for the reality. It wasn't some neat, linear pattern of stages. My experience wasn't a process that flowed or fit into a neat little circular chart that the experts designed. Instead, it was a chaotic storm of anxiety, depression, brain fog, humiliation, and self-disgust. The result left me wanting to hide under a rock and disappear.

Before going into rehab, I used to join the rooms of online AA meetings, listening to people share how amazing their sober lives were, and I'd feel…numb. I didn't believe sobriety could be real for me. It felt like they were talking about winning the lottery—something that happened to other people, not me.

But here I am now, telling *my* story. I wish I could share it with every struggling therapist out there. I want them to know that freedom and peace are possible. The joy I feel now isn't some elusive dream. It's real, and it's waiting for them, too.

Getting sober turned out to be the gateway to a life I couldn't have imagined. My days are now full of thrilling adventures, meaningful relationships, and new professional opportunities. Oh, and I didn't lose my license, by the way! My treatment met the requirements and, while the assessments weren't fun, they were a moment in time—now a moment in the past. What's more, my sobriety and growth has opened the door to even bigger ideas and dreams for helping others. The possibilities are endless!

Speaking of possibilities, I wonder if it is possible I'll survive the laser tag battle I'm about to have with the grandkids this afternoon. It's been a wild week, but it reminds me of what "living life to the fullest" really means. I'm so grateful I found the courage to reclaim my life and make it better than I honestly thought possible.

I wish you were here to join in the fun. Your laugh would fit in perfectly here. I know you'd be joining me in hilarious competitions with these youngsters. For now, imagine the love and laughter coming right through these letters. With a friendship like ours, you're never really that far away.

Sending my love,

- *L*

4. Where Healing Begins

Don't be jealous…but I just got back from Costa Rica, and it was amazing!

I stayed in a cabin right in the heart of the rainforest, surrounded by the hum of life, a world teeming with color, sound, and energy. Though it was hot and humid, the canopy of towering bamboo and flowering trees provided relief, offering a cool, dappled shade that made everything feel a little softer, a little dreamier.

On a guided jungle tour I took, it felt like I had stepped into a nature documentary. White-faced monkeys swung so close overhead that I could see their tiny fingers gripping the bark. Sloths clung lazily to the branches. Giant green iguanas sprawled like prehistoric kings on sun-warmed rocks. And the birds! Macaws, toucans, and countless others I didn't even know the names of painted the sky with flashes of color.

It was exhilarating—like being dropped into a brand-new world. This incredible adventure came as a bonus after attending a retreat in Costa Rica with a friend. I thought of you, knowing you would have loved the theme. It was rooted in both brain science and spiritual healing—exactly the kind of work we always geeked out over together.

The retreat center itself was like something out of a dream. Nestled in the lush Turrubares mountains near Jaco, everything was so intensely green it almost didn't seem real. Trees draped in moss, vines twisting like serpents, bamboo stalks as thick as pine trees. Flowers everywhere—from delicate lotuses in soft pinks and purples floating on the ponds, to bold, fiery birds of paradise stretching toward the sky.

And the wildlife? Let's just say I made some new jungle friends. I watched a "Jesus Christ" lizard sprint across the water, defying gravity on its hind legs. I listened to the symphony of the jungle—the layered trills of frogs, the rhythmic chirps of crickets, the occasional distant growl of something wild. There were only screens on the windows, so the sounds surrounded me completely, inescapable, immersive.

At first, I thought there was no way I would be able to sleep through it all. (You know all about my insomnia.) But I was wrong. I slept better than I have in years. Maybe it's true—maybe our bodies really do resonate with the sounds of nature. Maybe, for the first time in a long time, I was in harmony with something bigger than myself.

One night, as I lay there listening to the frogs, I remembered something my therapist told me years ago about addiction. She explained that when we sink into substance use disorder, we lose things in a specific order.

1. First, we lose our spiritual connection.
2. Then, we lose our emotional stability.
3. Finally, our physical bodies begin to break down.

Looking back, that was exactly how it happened for me.

Remember how you and I used to talk for hours about the mysteries of the universe, the depths of the soul, the unexplainable beauty of life? Over the course of my drinking, I can now see I lost all of that. I didn't just disconnect from my people—I disconnected from my higher power, which I comfortably call God.

Like so many alcoholics, I drank to escape. Escape emotions. Escape responsibilities. Escape relationships. Escape the relentless pressure of being the one who had it all together. And unfortunately, the escape didn't stop there. Without even realizing it, I was also escaping my connection to the divine.

I know we've talked so much about energy—the idea that everything vibrates at different frequencies, how we attract or repel things based on what we put out. And for me, alcohol seemed to dampen my vibration to the point that it was like trying to connect through a wall of pillows. Nothing got through. Not the presence I once felt so deeply with my source and creator. Not the loving comments from others. Not even friendships like ours.

And then there was the shame–the emotional earthquake that shook me to the core. Drinking compromised my morals, my judgment, my integrity. The little white lies stacked up like bricks in a wall between me and the people who cared about me. I hid my drinking. I missed commitments. I let people down. Each failure fed the shame, and the shame fueled more drinking.

It was a perfect, suffocating trap. Stability was a missing piece in my broken emotional world. And here's the cruel part—even love couldn't break through. You tried. Others tried. But I couldn't accept it. Because I didn't just dislike myself—I despised myself.

In this emotional turmoil, and the increased alcohol intake, my body broke down. There were more things wrong with me physiologically than I was aware of—from organs on their way to disease to compromised brain functioning, I was a biological mess.

The good news is that the way addiction dismantles a person is also the way we put ourselves back together–albeit in reverse order.

1. First, my body had to heal.
2. Then, my emotional stability returned.
3. And finally, I found my way back to a healthy spiritual connection.

My physical healing led the way. Detox. Rehab. Proper nutrition. Exercise. Neurotherapy. Rebuilding from the inside out. Little by little, as my body healed, my mind followed. Too often, our society tries to heal in the wrong order, and it is set up to fail. For decades, people believed SUD (substance use disorder) was just a psychological disorder based on trauma, and sufferers were sent to mental institutions where they rarely recovered. Even today, many professionals mistakenly conclude that a patient needs to heal their trauma first so they won't *need* to drink. But too often, that process stirs up intense emotional pain, reactivates traumatic memories, and evokes more desperation ultimately overwhelming the client and rarely leading to successful recovery. What is truly needed is an efficient and compassionate detox, followed by a rehabilitation program (ideally at least 30 days), to prepare the body for the next steps of healing. For me, the healing was a slow process. After I got through the detox phase, I knew I was continually moving forward, but sometimes the progress was barely noticeable. I felt vulnerable and tender—if not guarded—for quite a while. But eventually, as my body continued to get stronger and healthier, my emotions felt less jumbled. I leaned on my therapy groups, friends, and family, even when it was hard to face the difficult and painful feelings.

Addiction recovery is a messy process, leaving pieces of one's being scattered across time and space. With continued healing, the pieces do eventually come back together, but the whole is not what it was before. I don't think there's a final "arrival point" with emotional or spiritual healing. It's a lifelong journey.

But I stayed committed to the process—therapy, intensive outpatient, support groups, hard conversations with my family. I did everything I could to repair the damage I had done because, at the end of the day, we are communal beings. We heal in connection, not in isolation.

And finally came my spiritual healing. That one is harder for me to define. I don't think I ever fully lost my connection to God, but it was sporadic, unreliable—like a radio signal cutting in and out. Sometimes, it seemed like someone had put the central tenets of my faith through one of those voice-changing toys, distorting the message until it was unrecognizable.

But in Costa Rica, I heard it and felt it clearly again. For me, spiritual messages often come through nature. The towering trees, the endless chorus of creatures, the waves gently rocking me in the crystal-clear waters of the ocean. It was all love. It was all a reminder that I belong–that I am part of something vast, and miraculous, and alive. I was reminded of what's always been true: even in my darkest moments, I was never alone.

I wish you could've been there with me soaking it all in, finding that same peace. I know you would have enjoyed it, as I did. I hope I never forget the feeling of being embraced by not just the ocean, or the jungle, but by the Divine of the universe.

For now, I'll leave you with this quote from Rumi I know you'll appreciate: "You are not a drop in the ocean. You are the ocean in a drop."

As always, sending my love.

- *L*

5. Glass Frogs

Did you know there are frogs so transparent you can see their heart beating inside them? I didn't—not until I saw one up close in Central America. These tiny, living glass frogs are no more than two inches long with a bright lime green on their backs, but their underbellies are completely clear. If you hold one gently in your hand, you can see its delicate organs—the red of its heart, the white of its intestines, and pinkish grey of its other organs.

Imagine if we humans had that kind of transparency. Once you stop laughing—or gasping—imagine how cool it would be if we could see the miracle of our insides!

Actually, I think of how helpful it could have been if, just by looking at me, someone could have seen my liver turning toxic, my gut lining deteriorating, my brain being damaged and hijacked by alcohol. But of course, we don't have that luxury. The damage is hidden beneath our skin for a long time.

I didn't realize how much danger I was in until I got to rehab and they ran my bloodwork. I remember sitting there, exhausted and detoxing, when the doctor told me I was on the verge of permanent liver damage. I had no symptoms—at least none I was willing to acknowledge. I wasn't yellow. I wasn't doubled over in pain. I could still function most days. I told myself I was fine, but I wasn't fine.

Hearing those results sent a shock through me, but it wasn't totally unfamiliar. I had seen this story play out before—just not in my own body. My father suffered from cirrhosis, failing kidneys, and a body wrecked by alcoholism. He was in constant pain, slowly deteriorating until he chose to end his own life. I knew how his story ended, but I had convinced myself that mine would be different. That I was different. Turns out, I wasn't.

I sometimes think about how close I came to my own point of no return. The moment when the damage becomes irreversible, when healing is no longer an option. I don't know where that line is, and honestly, I don't want to find out. What I do know is that, despite everything I put my body through, it still fought for me. The moment I gave it what it needed instead of poisoning it, it started working to repair itself.

When I learned in rehab just how bad my liver was, I panicked. I wasn't ready to die. So, I went into full research mode, talking to doctors, reading studies, and hunting for anything that might help. The medical center wouldn't allow me to take supplements I didn't come in with during those first thirty days, but I still had control over what I ate and put into my body.

I remember standing in the cafeteria, staring at my food options like my life depended on them—because, in a way, it did. I know you're probably grinning, imagining me fine-tuning my "menu" in a rehab buffet!

In my research, I had learned that chronic alcohol use often leads to hypoglycemia—and during recovery, blood sugar crashes can trigger strong cravings for alcohol as the body looks for a quick energy fix. Isn't that fascinating? Fueled by this insight, I switched to a hypoglycemic diet to balance my blood sugar and give my body it's best fighting chance. My mornings started with one cup of black coffee, one or two halves of grapefruit with just a touch of honey, and handfuls of fresh berries: blueberries, blackberries, and raspberries. (The acidity was said to be good for liver function.) Sometimes I added oatmeal with nuts and cranberries. Lunch included spinach and leafy green salads piled with fresh veggies, sunflower seeds, olives, avocado, and extra olive oil with the dressing. I wanted those healthy fats to further aid the healing process. Dinners consisted of lean proteins with fresh vegetables. I avoided all processed sugars, bread/gluten, starches, and most dairy.

It sounds simple, right? Maybe even boring. But within two weeks, my blood panel showed astonishing improvement. The doctors were amazed and shared they hadn't seen such a turnaround in so little time. My liver was no longer in immediate danger!

I almost couldn't believe it. After years of poisoning myself, my body was already healing. It was a relief—and a revelation. It showed me the power of education, discipline, and the body's resilience.

Unfortunately, my liver damage was only one aspect of the total harm done to my body. My gut was wrecked. My kidneys were strained. And here's the real kicker—I was significantly malnourished. That truly was a shock. I wasn't underweight. In fact, I had been carrying extra weight for years, so it never occurred to me that my body wasn't absorbing nutrients. But it turns out, no matter how many "superfood" smoothies I drank, my body couldn't process the vitamins or minerals because the alcohol was interfering with absorption. My system was so compromised that I was slowly starving at a cellular level.

I had convinced myself that I was being "proactive" about my health. Sure, I drank too much, but I was taking my vitamins and eating my greens to counter the alcohol intake and keep myself in check. It was a deception I had told myself so many times that I believed it. But the truth was there, hiding under the surface, just waiting to be revealed.

There's so much basic, life-saving information like this that people don't know—especially those still drinking and using. I wish I could share it with everyone, especially those who have no idea what's happening inside them.

I think about those glass frogs, so perfectly transparent. They don't have to wonder if they're okay—they just are. Of course, they also don't put poison in their bodies, lie to themselves, or pretend everything is fine while secretly dying inside. Maybe that's the lesson. Not to live in fear of what's hidden, but to find a way to stop doing things you would want to hide in the first place.

If I had the sense of a frog, I wouldn't have needed blood tests to tell me whether or not I was okay. Maybe I'll make that my new motto: "Just have the sense of a frog." With that, I too, could avoid putting things in my body or practicing behaviors that are destructive to my health—to my being.

Thanks for continuing to be my listening ear, even when I can't sit with you face to face. Know that I am hugging you with my heart and sending my love...

- *L*

P.S. You were always so good at motivating people to take action—I wish I had your brain and gift of inspiring others to get the word out about this stuff!

6. Turtles and Truths

Aloha! Yes, I'm speaking Hawaiian as I am just returning from a fabulous retreat in Maui.

Remember how we used to dream of going to Hawaii together and attending a real luau? The mainland parties our friends put on were fun, but we dreamed of being where the real hula and fire dancers showed off their stuff! I didn't make it to any luaus on this trip, but I also have no regrets.

Instead, I just soaked up all the crazy beauty around me. The royal blue ocean that glittered and crashed. The brilliant greenery and brightly colored flowers that came to life in every direction I looked. It felt like a present day *Garden of Eden*.

While the retreat classes were at a cool eco-retreat center inland, you know me, I still spent most of my time on the beach or in the ocean. Smelling the fresh salty air with floral hints, along with the hum and rhythm of the waves, provided a gentle reminder that I, too, was allowed to flow and change.

There were so many sea turtles. Some of them were huge! There was actually a breaker wall that I thought was made of boulders, only to realize upon closer look, it was covered with as many turtles as rocks. Even swimming in the ocean, there were a couple of times I actually saw them catching the waves with me. It was spectacular.

The retreat's theme of finding and living from "Your Authentic Self" appealed to me as I have needed to remember and redefine who I am after years of being lost in my alcoholism. The beautiful and tranquil setting didn't hurt either (as if I needed an excuse to go)! I imagine the laughter and fun we would have had if you could have been there with me.

It turned out the topic we worked on most at the retreat was shame. That's really when I knew I was right where I needed to be. I felt like shame had chewed me up and spit me out during the painful process of addiction, rehab, and if I'm honest, sometimes even recovery. Because shame has a way of disguising my reality, of confusing the facts, it has often been hard to make sense of my life.

It was enlightening to recognize how shame inhibits us from living authentically. It stunts our growth in ways I hadn't realized before, by keeping us frightened and therefore hiding from potential opportunities. I know it kept me from putting myself out there, not wanting to show vulnerability or emotion, as I worried others would see me as I saw myself: an imposter pretending to be a good and capable person, with deep flaws and "unlovable parts" of my being lurking just beneath a shiny surface.

Shame isn't just something we feel—it's something that sticks, that clings to us like the weight of the ocean's current, pulling us back every time we try to move forward. It convinces us that we are not good enough, that we will always be less than others. But the truth is, it's a lie, and letting go of that burden is where the real work begins.

Shame skews our perception and hooks us into judgement, comparison, perfectionism, and feelings of unworthiness. I have been up close and personal with all of these. I had always kind of melded together the concepts of shame and guilt, but when guilt was defined as doing something that is out of alignment with my value system, I started to notice a nuanced difference. The feeling of guilt alerts me to something I would want to make amends for or try to make right. Shame, on the other hand, is the feeling that I don't just make mistakes or do bad things, I actually *am* a mistake. "I am bad." With that message in your head, of course you don't want to acknowledge any mistakes. And in that way, shame actually gets in the way of us becoming our truest and best self.

Like many sufferers of SUD I've known, I do believe shame fed my addiction, and addiction fed my shame. Feelings of unworthiness and being unlovable started early in my life, as early as I can remember. Of course, there is more to this story, like the abuse and trauma I suffered early on, but that's for another letter. The point is, even though my alcohol use and SUD didn't come onto the scene until mid-life, I know these negative core beliefs certainly contributed to my "drinking as a solution." While there is definitely a massive biological component to my alcohol addiction, the psychological pieces have also played a big role. The shame was already there, but the addiction also fed it, and both grew.

31

If I were still drinking, I think I still would have enjoyed the retreat, but permanent healing, growth, and change would have definitely been hampered. Sure, I was able to go days or even a week without drinking before I went to rehab, but I know there was both guilt and shame around my drinking that would have prevented healthy processing with others on a deeper level if I had gone to a retreat like this years ago.

Instead, my mind was clear, and my heart was open enough to receive and practice these teachings. Believe it or not, I really started believing the truth that I am worthy just because I exist. For most of my life I have believed *in theory* that I am lovable and loved, but now this honestly feels different—like it's not something theoretically true, but something I *know*.

For so long, I felt like I was adrift, disconnected from the world and everyone in it. My addiction kept me isolated—physically and emotionally—and I couldn't sustain any real connections. Now, though, life and relationships are more than I ever imagined they could be. These friendships, these genuine bonds, have become the foundation of my healing. I feel more whole, more capable of helping others, and dare I say it—more me.

I wish you could meet these new friends of mine, I think you'd fit right in. For now, know that I'm sending my love, as always, and thinking of you every step of the way.

- *L*

7. Seen

You have always been that amazing friend who I felt really saw me. Not just the me I showed the world, but the real me. The one beneath the surface. You always seemed to see past my reactions, my carefully curated expressions, straight into something deeper—something truer, something beautiful.

It has not been easy for me to allow myself to be seen. In fact, it has been one of my hardest challenges in life because it requires vulnerability, courage, and trust.

And I didn't learn those things growing up. I learned that vulnerability wasn't safe. That sharing my emotions, especially the hard ones, often led to dismissal, discomfort, or outright rejection. If I was upset, I was told to stop overreacting. If I was sad, I was reminded why I shouldn't be. If I cried, people either mocked me or pulled away.

There wasn't space for my emotions in my home. There was already too much emotion, too much volatility, too much fighting, too much chaos. And so, like a sponge, I absorbed the energy of those around me. But what I absorbed, I had no idea how to process.

So, I did what I saw others do. I learned to mask it. To put on a happy face, to think positively, to present well. That's how people liked me. That's how I fit in. And for a while, it worked.

It was always funny to me how often people would compliment me for being caring, kind, and emotionally in tune—only to, at other times, criticize me for being too sensitive. Apparently, being emotionally aware was only acceptable when it made others comfortable.

So, I kept it all inside. For years. For decades.

The problem was that this strategy was slowly starving me. By not allowing myself to be vulnerable with others, I robbed myself of the very thing I needed most: connection. My inability to show up fully kept people at a distance, and worse, it kept them from feeling like they could be real with me, too.

It is nearly impossible to be truly loved when you can't engage in honest interaction. Because to be fully loved, you must be seen.

John O'Donohue describes it beautifully in *Eternal Echoes*:

> Vulnerability is an infinitely precious thing. There is nothing as lonely as that which has become hardened. When your heart hardens, your life has become numb.

And isn't that the truth?

I used to think that hardening myself was the safest choice. That keeping people at a comfortable distance would protect me. That if I just numbed the bad, I could escape the pain.

But as Brené Brown says, "We cannot selectively numb emotions, when we numb the painful emotions, we also numb the positive emotions."

And that's exactly what I did. I numbed myself with alcohol. I numbed the pain of rejection. I numbed the fear of being "too much" or "not enough." I numbed the loneliness, the insecurity, the exhaustion of always performing my way through life. And in the process, I also numbed the joy, the love, the deep, meaningful connection I so desperately wanted but didn't know how to reach for.

Thankfully, that's not the end of my story. Getting sober forced me to step into vulnerability in ways I never had before. Recovery demanded honesty—not just with others, but also with myself. It asked me to take off the mask, to stop pretending, to let myself be seen, even in my most broken state.

And you know what happened? I didn't disappear. I didn't break. I didn't shatter into a million irreparable pieces. I healed.

I'm still healing. I'm still learning to be vulnerable, to show up fully, to let people see me as I really am. But I am here. Present. Open. Alive. And I am learning to believe that I am enough—just as I am.

So again, thank you for seeing me. For not looking away. For making space for my messy, imperfect, beautiful self. It's friends like you, the ones who've held my hand along this journey, that make this life doable.

Sending my love,

- *L*

8. Brownie Cake

Okay, so I have another funny story for you. I think I told you our daughter was getting married (which she did, and it was beautiful). But did I tell you I was making her wedding cake—in Costa Rica!? Well, as it turns out, I actually made wedding brownies.

I had this whole vision planned out—gorgeous, rich chocolate brownies, tiered beautifully on a five-layer stand I'd ordered from Etsy. And what better place to make them than at a resort that had its own cocoa farm and made its own chocolate? I mean, this felt like a perfect plan—fated to be glorious.

But fate, as it turns out, has a mischievous sense of humor.

I had brought all my own pans and supplies, other than ingredients, which I was sure I could get onsite. When I went to get some cocoa powder from the resort, however, I was told they didn't have any. At a cocoa farm. No unsweetened cocoa, no powdered form, nothing. My options? Either drive two hours into the city (which there wasn't nearly enough time for) or get creative.

Someone suggested seeing if the resort offered ceremonial cacao. I had no idea what that was, but I was out of options. So I asked, they said yes, and just like that, I was committed to making wedding brownies with an ingredient I'd never used before!

What followed was an adventure in culinary improvisation. I researched recipes, made some calculations, and threw together a plan that was part science, part sheer hope. There was no time for a test run—it was go-time.

I asked the cooks to preheat the oven to 350°F. They just smiled and shook their heads. Apparently, they had no way of knowing what temperature they were baking at! However, these cooks used the oven daily, and while they had never heard of brownies before (can you believe it?), I just asked them to cook the brownies like they would a cake.

A small team of us chopped and grated cacao bars, then melted butter, sugar, and cacao together over a makeshift double boiler (which was really

36

just two odd-sized pans precariously stacked on the stove in this third-world type kitchen setting). When the batter was ready, we poured it into the pan, and into the oven it went. Somehow, miraculously, the first batch turned out great. (Whew!) So, we made more.

The second batch? A little undercooked—probably because we baked two large pans at once. After all, it was crunch time! Fortunately, the consistency was good enough and they still tasted great, so we moved on. Because we were so up against the clock, the last batch we baked was still in the oven while the cooks were preparing lunch for resort guests.

When I opened the oven, instead of rich chocolate, I was hit with the overwhelming smell of garlic. I realized the cooks were baking the brownies with everything they were serving for lunch, including savory vegetables and garlic bread! My wedding brownies had been cohabitating with an entire buffet.

I was curious what they would end up tasting like. Had they absorbed the scents of the lunch foods? Would my daughter's wedding brownies taste like garlic and veggies? I gave the brownies a little extra time in the oven to try and compensate for all the other items baking in there with them, but everything was a total guess.

In the end, my daughter's wedding brownies turned out wonderfully despite the guessing game I was playing all morning!

Making these brownies felt a lot like my early days of recovery: unsure, improvisational, and sometimes a bit messy. When I started out, I really had no idea how to do this. In fact, there were several serious attempts before going into rehab—even with professional help—that didn't work long term. So, the adventure of recovery was a day-to-day challenge. Everyone had different ideas or suggestions. Everyone had a different experience with a different set of circumstances. In essence, they each shared their own recipe for staying sober, and no two were exactly the same.

When it was my own experience, all I could do was make my best educated guesses and move forward. And each time I pulled out a batch of "brownies" that didn't look right, I remembered the cooks in the kitchen who knew the oven better than I did. My sponsor, spiritual teachers, and fellow travelers in recovery have been the steady hands that helped me adjust the temperature when it felt like everything was burning or undercooked. They reminded me not to give up when the recipe seemed all wrong.

Fortunately, the most recent "batches" in my recovery have been successful, which has given me valuable information on how to move further along that pathway. But every now and then, I have an experience that is like pulling out brownies that just don't look or smell quite right.

Sometimes this can even send me spiraling into a place of doubt or fear. A couple of these dark experiences have caused me to think about reaching for the bottle, even after months or years of sobriety. However, by accepting the support of others with wisdom and experience, I've continued to move forward in recovery.

I hear your voice in my head telling me to "never give up." There isn't one clear or standard recipe for attaining and maintaining sobriety. Sometimes, we find ourselves forced to improvise through creative endeavors. While I believe all life experiences can be good for us in some way, as they are all opportunities for growth and perspective, I am so happy the brownies of my recovery journey are a sweet-tasting success, today.

So, with that in mind, when my next awkward moment arrives, I will say with confidence, "I'll have another brownie, please. Give me the garlic one with a side of veggies."

- *L*

9. The Healing Frequency

I am doing the most exciting thing! You know how I've always been into music? Well, this year I've embarked on a new adventure with something called "sound healing." It all started after I broke my ankle and had to be non-weight bearing for two months. That was a long time for me to sit still, so naturally, I found a way to turn my forced rest into something new and interesting. I signed up for an online course and proceeded to collect a full set of crystal singing bowls—because, you know, *go big or go home*.

I've always known music was powerful, but I didn't fully grasp *how* powerful until I dove into this world of sound therapy. Our brains and bodies are, at their core, frequency-based systems. Sound is just one of the many ways we interact with frequencies in our environment. For example, neurostimulation works by delivering specific frequencies to the brain, helping to regulate neural activity. Scents (like essential oils) operate through frequency-based signals that our olfactory system translates into physiological responses. Light therapy—whether it's the blue light that affects our sleep cycles or red light used for healing—also operates on specific wavelengths that interact with the body. And then there are binaural beats, where two slightly different sound frequencies in each ear create a third, perceived frequency in the brain that can promote relaxation, focus, or even altered states of consciousness.

Though its origins are unclear (often attributed to Einstein), this quote holds a truth that echoes through my being:

> We are slowed down sound and light waves, a walking bundle of frequencies tuned into the music of the cosmos. We are souls dressed up in sacred biochemical garments, and our bodies are the instruments through which our souls play their music.

When I place a singing bowl on or near someone's body and play it, the vibrations move through their tissues and cells, much like how ultrasound waves are used in medical imaging or how focused sound waves can break up kidney stones. It's science *and* it's ancient wisdom—both Western medicine and Eastern traditions, like Traditional Chinese Medicine and Ayurveda, which have long understood that energy, sound, and frequency play a role in healing.

I recently added a set of authentic seven-metal Tibetan singing bowls to my collection, and wow, do they take things to a whole new level! The harmonies they produce are rich and complex, and the vibrations can be felt deep in the body. I continue playing my Native American flutes, along with various chimes and drums, which makes for quite a fun setup. Basically, I've become a one-woman orchestra of potential healing vibrations.

And the most incredible part? I'm seeing real results.

A woman recently came to one of my sound healing events after suffering for three months with an illness that no treatment seemed to touch. She had seen doctors, taken medication, tried alternative therapies, but nothing worked. After the session, she told me she felt something *shift*. She wasn't sure what it was, but for the first time in months, she felt relief. And the next day? Her symptoms were completely gone. Just like that.

Now, I'm not saying I have magical powers (though I'd gladly take them if offered). What I *am* saying is that sound has an incredible capacity to interact with the body in ways we don't fully understand yet. And the research is there—sound, music, and vibration affect us in profound ways.

Music is processed in the amygdala, the same part of the brain that plays a role in emotion and memory. This is why certain songs can bring back vivid memories or change our mood in an instant. Listening to pleasurable music activates the brain's reward system, increasing dopamine levels—something that's especially beneficial for those recovering from substance use, and others whose dopamine systems are dysregulated. Playing or singing music together also releases oxytocin, the bonding hormone, and this is why we feel connected when we sing in a choir, drum in a group, or even hum along with someone else.

I think sound healing, and many of these frequency-based therapies, can be really beneficial in the recovery process. After years of substance use, the brain is often left depleted of dopamine, oxytocin, and other vital neurotransmitters that regulate mood, motivation, and emotional well-being. That's why early recovery can feel *flat*—because the brain is trying to recalibrate. Sound healing offers a non-invasive, natural way to stimulate the brain's reward pathways, helping to rebuild the circuits that have been damaged by a substance use disorder.

Calming frequencies help regulate the nervous system, shifting it from a state of fight-or-flight (which many in recovery struggle with) to a state of relaxation and balance. This is why so many people report feeling deeply relaxed, grounded, and even euphoric after sound healing sessions. It's a way to reconnect with the body, quiet the mind, and create a sense of peace that doesn't require external substances.

On top of all this, sound healing works deeply with energy centers in the body, often referred to as chakras. While chakras are not something you can see on an MRI, they closely align with physiological systems, particularly the endocrine system and nervous system.

For example:

- The heart chakra—which governs love, connection, and emotional balance—is centered around the physical heart, an

organ that contains approximately 40,000 neurons (yes, your heart literally has its own mini-brain!).
- The solar plexus chakra, associated with personal power and gut instinct, corresponds with the enteric nervous system, which contains about 500 million neurons and is often called "the second brain."

So, when people talk about sound balancing chakras, it's not just an abstract concept—it's a physiological process, influencing both the nervous and endocrine systems in measurable ways.

I love learning about this because, honestly, it all makes *sense*. We feel music and sound in our bodies, whether it's the way a deep bass vibrates in our chest, or the way a gentle melody soothes our nerves. And now I get to bring that experience to others. It's healing for *them*, and it's healing for *me*.

Maybe I'll write a book about all this someday, but for now, I'm just enjoying the process.

I'll leave you with this poem I love, by Hafiz:

> I am a hole in a flute that the Christ's breath moves through—listen to this music.
>
> I am the concert from the movement of every creature singing in myriad chords.
>
> And every dancer, their foot I know and lift.
>
> And every brush and hand, well, that is me too, who caresses any canvas or cheek.
>
> How did I become all these things, and beyond all things?
>
> It was my destiny, as it is yours. My poems are about our glorious journey.

We are a hole in a flute, a moment in space, that the
Christ's body can move through and sway

All forms—in an exquisite dance—as the wind in a
forest.

Goodnight, dear friend. I'm singing a lullaby to you in my heart and
sending my love...

- *L*

10. Desert Wisdom

Have you ever been to New Mexico? I went last week for the first time, and it was an incredible experience! I was in the Chama Canyon which has the same type of high desert beauty as Sedona, AZ, with the painted sandstone hills. It was so peaceful, and I enjoyed spending hours by the Chama River playing my singing bowls and flutes.

As you might have guessed by now, I take my sound healing tools seriously, but it's okay if you laugh at this story. I was sitting in my camping chair beside the river, playing one of my flutes, when out of the corner of my eye, I saw something small and dark scurry out of the bushes. My eyes quickly darted to the spot—not ten feet away, and what did I see? A black, hairy tarantula, about three inches in diameter, crossing the path and heading straight for me! I tried to keep playing as though I didn't notice him, but he walked straight up to my foot. He probably would have kept going right up my leg or into my bag if I didn't startle and jump! I quickly pulled out my camera to get a picture of him, and he reared up, thrashing his legs until I backed off. Then, in an instant, he just turned around and went back into the bushes.

The next day, while exploring the canyon in my jeep, I noticed a large, shiny rattlesnake coiled up in the middle of the road. I drove around it, but when I returned several hours later, it was still in the same place. You know me, the curious one. I couldn't help it. I stopped my jeep on the shoulder and got out. There was no one else around, so I could hear the tiny pebbles under my hiking boots with every step as I walked across the pavement very slowly. Was it alive? I stepped closer. As I approached, it silently did that thing snakes do with their tongues. I probably should have turned around at this point, but I wondered if it was injured…so I moved a little closer, still. Then, breaking the silence, it suddenly shook its fancy black rattler, and I knew that whatever its condition, I had tempted fate enough…I let it be and backed away slowly until I was safely inside the jeep.

Most humans perceive these fascinating creatures as threatening "unlovelies" in the animal kingdom. It seems we have an unspoken hierarchy for what we deem beautiful or lovable, but I believe that all life is sacred and amazing.

Maybe I wanted to serenade a tarantula and visit with a rattlesnake because I've felt judged in a similar way, being an alcoholic, going into rehab, and even sometimes now in recovery. Everybody knows a story about someone who suffered because of a drunk driver or some other horrendous act where substances were involved. I still imagine others looking at me like I am somehow that broken, flawed—even dangerous—part of society. That I am the "unlovely" nobody wants to get too close to.

So often, the truth is opposite of what we fear. Do you know what many Native American cultures believe about the totem wisdom of the tarantula? They believe spiders are spiritual teachers and carriers of wisdom. They say the spider teaches us to maintain a balance—between past and future, physical and spiritual, male and female. Spider wisdom tells us that everything we do in the present is weaving what we will encounter in the future. Due to its unique characteristics, the spider has even come to be associated with magic and the energy of creation. It is a symbol of creative power.

As for the rattlesnake, it is believed to symbolize protection, strength, and resilience. Its ability to shed its skin represents renewal and transformation. Its rattling sound warns of danger, serving as a reminder to stay vigilant and aware of one's surroundings. Additionally, the rattlesnake's connection to the earth and its ability to sense vibrations in the soil symbolize grounding and intuition.

In the same way, people who struggle with substance use disorders are not always what one might think. There is even research suggesting most individuals who struggle with substance use disorders are not only incredibly intelligent, but also deeply caring, highly sensitive, and often remarkably creative with a playful spirit. People like you and me aren't flawed at the core. In fact, we are likely gifted! We aren't members of a degenerate, lower class of society that should be feared because of some weakness or immoral character flaw. We are merely sufferers of a disease that sometimes hides or distorts our best qualities.

I can hear you now, encouraging me, and I thank you. Know that I've always believed in your goodness, as well. Your friendship shows me the value of having the support of other sufferers who truly understand. Only one who has "walked a mile in these hiking boots" really could.

- *L*

11. *The Worm and the Apple*

It's 11 a.m., and the tea kettle is whistling. It's time for tea and cookies. This was a special ritual for the last several years, until my mom passed in December. I remember when you joined us for this delightful practice a couple years ago during the holidays. That was a sweet time. My eyes are leaking and my heart aches as I think of and miss you both right now.

Anyone who knew my mom knew how much she loved her teatime. And anyone who was close to her has a story to tell of a special conversation or activity done around this precious ceremony.

When mom still lived in her home, I remember these sweet breaks together outside on her deck in Santa Barbara. It was a sad day when things changed after her terrible fall. For several months, we didn't know if she would even survive, as my brother, sister, and I took turns flying out to California to care for her. Thankfully, she did recover, but it was clear she could no longer live alone, so she came to live with my husband and me in Colorado.

While it was an honor and a blessing to be her full-time caregiver for a while, it was also really challenging. Her fall was at the very beginning of the Covid pandemic, so everything and everyone was in a state of crisis. I remember you and me talking about how tough it was to be therapists during this time, trying to calm and comfort our clients while struggling with many of the same feelings, ourselves. Add to this the sad fact that for the first half of those three years, I was in the worst season of my alcoholism.

Don't get me wrong. Mom and I did have many precious moments during that time. But our tea and cookie time conversations often included her probing, like, "Are you okay? Is there anything I can do to help?" Her love and concern were sweet, but also annoying to me at the time. Some part of me knew she could see what I was trying to hide. Her subtle questions were calling my bluff, and my defenses only grew. Some days, her unofficial accountability would help me avoid drinking for a while. Other days, I just didn't care.

In comparison, after I got sober, we had so many uncompromised precious times together. So many amazing, deep conversations. We would explore ideas and possibilities together, seeing everyday life as miraculous. We would encourage one another to be the best we can be in whatever circumstance we might find ourselves. (Much like the front porch talks you and I used to have.)

Looking back now, I can see how my mom was offering her fruit of love and encouragement, as I suppose only a mom can do, while also trying to cultivate the best of what she knew to be within me—somewhere.

I have recently been reminded, by an apple tree in the yard no less, that we are all created to bear whatever fruit we are capable of offering to others. Though it was autumn and most of the other apples had already fallen or been harvested, this one, small red apple remained on a nearly leafless branch. When I got closer, thinking I would pick it, I noticed it had become a nice comfy home for a big, juicy worm. (How "human" of me to assume the tree's fruit was offered only to me.)

In any case, when it comes to offering my own gifts, I'll seek to do it just as the apple tree did. I'll aim to simply make what I have available to whoever wishes to receive it, with no strings attached. I'm learning I don't need to force anything on others or lace my "fruit" with expectations, as you are aware I have been known to do. I will just put it out there and let whatever happens from there happen.

When I'm with clients in my office, I think I'm actually pretty good at being present, listening, and offering encouragement for ways they can help themselves. After all, it is what good therapists are supposed to do— offer our fruits of encouragement and insights and let the client do with it what they will. However, I recognize I'm not always so good at doing this outside of my professional role or beyond the comfort of my clinical office.

As a fellow helper, I'm sure you won't be surprised by this—it is much easier for me to offer my fruitful help than it is to allow myself to receive help from others. It's even more difficult for me to ask for it.

That worm in the last red apple reminded me that I also need to be willing to use my "spiritual hands" to harvest and gather the fruit others have to offer. I think this is what my mother was trying to help me with as she encouraged and nurtured me, to bring my best to the surface with her questions and her enduring kindness.

As I reflect on this, I'm working now to offer myself grace and forgiveness for ways of the past. I will simply set the intention to keep my heart open, giving love without expectation and actively receiving it in return. I will offer my "apples" to whomever can receive them—human or worm. Both are okay.

Wish you were beside me right now to do a gift exchange! You were always so good at helping me practice goals like these. For now, I will practice in remembrance of my mom—and you—doing as Thich Nach Hanh instructs: "Bear fruit, but also use your hands for harvest. And everything you do, do it for love's sake." Now, if you'll excuse me, I'm going to take a few minutes to enjoy the rest of my tea and cookies!

As always, sending my love...

- *L*

12. After the Flames

I was thinking about you today while I went on this stunning hike outside of Hamilton, Montana. I truly miss the adventurous walks we used to take together. I felt a strong urge to get back out into nature as it's still where I feel most connected to God, as well as all life. Plus, great beauty abounds in the Bitterroot Valley in early October. On this hike through the woods to Blodgett Trail Overlook, the colors were astounding. The yellows, greens, oranges, and reds of the leaves against the backdrop of the bright blue sky created a vibrant stage for all the wildlife scurrying around, preparing for winter.

The woods were filled with many different types of trees, both deciduous and evergreen. As I walked along the dirt trail, I noticed that interspersed with healthy trees of all sizes were lots of trees partly charred by a recent forest fire. There were also quite a few fallen, long-dead trees scattered throughout. In some areas, there were literally thousands of young trees crowded together, each seeming to compete to be one of the few survivors that would make it to adulthood.

I came upon a placard that told hikers about a recent wildfire, and it specifically described all the benefits a forest reaps after such destruction. It told how the rubbish gets burned away, and the trees that are burned become hollows for nature to do her magic, attracting insects, birds, and animals that are crucial to the overall health of the forest's ecosystem.

Standing in front of the placard, my chest and shoulders tightened...I couldn't help but reflect on what initially felt like the destruction of my life a few short years ago. When my life seemed to be falling apart, and especially when I finally surrendered to getting help, it felt like a wildfire of sorts was tearing through all that I thought was important and valuable. With relief, and dare I say joy, I see how it all turned out to be the creation of a new beginning.

You know me and my imagination. Standing on that path, I saw all the fallen dead trees around me as the ancestors who had come before me. It was like a physical representation of how I am part of a larger familial, human ecosystem in which I march forward with all the residual blessings and curses of generations past.

I then squinted as I turned to all the baby trees packed together in a small sunlit patch where the forest canopy had been burned away. I felt sadness and grief as I reflected on how most of them wouldn't survive. As in much of nature, it truly would end up being the survival of the fittest. Only the strongest saplings in the best positions to receive sun and rain—without too much exposure to the harsh winter winds or diseases—would grow to be full-sized, adult trees.

I found myself frozen there as tears began to well in my eyes. Grief rushed over me, and even despair for a moment, as I thought of all the people suffering from addiction this year who literally won't survive the disease. I read recently that, like too many young trees with a world of potential, there are currently over forty million people in the U.S. struggling with a substance use disorder. Apparently, only about five percent of those receive any treatment at all, and only one percent gets *adequate* treatment for their condition. Of those who get help, only about eighteen percent stay sober in the first year, and only half of those who make it to their second year of sobriety stay that way for the long term.

The statistics are flabbergasting, because we have so much available to us these days, especially here in the States. Part of the problem, for me, is that most rehab programs don't provide a well-rounded bio-psycho-social-spiritual approach. By that, I mean a program that includes adequate and appropriate medications integrated with good talk therapy (alone and in groups), something therapeutic for the body, and a spiritually conscious support system. The one percent of rehabilitation programs that do offer the whole package are outrageously expensive, and insurance often refuses to cover them.

Don't even get me started about the $35,000 out of pocket I had to pay to get my help at an effective rehab center for just one month. I wiped out my savings, borrowed from retirement, and had to set up a three-year payment plan. Even after I had resigned myself to the fact that I needed help, this overwhelming financial barrier kept me from going into full treatment for over a year. It is one of the top excuses to put off rehab, and realistically a valid one, for most people. Instead of taking the plunge, most sufferers of

SUD (like me) just keep trying harder and failing harder as they attempt to get sober on their own.

Just at the edge of the little clearing packed with saplings, I saw a tall pine tree with two tops. One was charred and piece-by-piece sending its spent branches to the forest floor. The other seemed to be waving its healthy dark green needles in the wind at me, as it continued to reach toward the sky. I smiled a little as I thought maybe that tree represents me. Not only did going to rehab literally save my life, it also created a better *quality* of life than I imagined was possible for me. Even if I could have stopped drinking on my own, I would have missed out on so many supportive, educational, and healing experiences that have helped me do more than just stay sober. Today, I am so grateful for choosing a high-quality treatment facility. I'm grateful for the care I was given. I'm grateful for the loving support of family and friends, along with the wonderful recovery groups and resources I connected with. Mostly, I am grateful to be one of the survivors.

As I was getting close to the final outlook on the trail today, a dad came walking down with his two young children. The little boy's face lit up with a big smile as he piped up and told me, "When you get to the top, it's a really pretty view!" I smiled back and thought, *I kind of expected as much, with it being such a popular trail, you know!* However, when I got to that overlook, the beauty was beyond what I could have imagined.

Looking to the right, there were steep, rocky cliffs in beautiful grey-blue and purple hues, dotted with the contrasting warm colors of turning leaves and brush sprinkled here and there. To my left was the side of the mountain I had just climbed, still vibrant with greens, yellows, and reds. Straight across the valley was the town, nestled low in the valley. It looked quaint, yet spread out, with a wide river running all the way through.

Words can't adequately describe this spectacular view. I felt lighter and freer there, on top of the world. Honestly, my friend, it's not that different from the immense freedom and joy I feel living with sobriety after suffering for years in the bondage of addiction. What's more, I can now see and appreciate my own beautiful new growth as a person, appreciating all I have survived—and overcome. While I would have loved sharing this wonderful experience with you in person, I will just imagine you into the beautiful scene instead!

Sending you my love, with mountainous echoes...

- *L*

13. *The Fire Within*

I can imagine your smirk as I tell you about this recent experience I had. I know it's not really in your wheelhouse or belief system, and that's okay. But it was really significant for me, and I trust you, so I want to share about it anyway.

A few weeks ago, I participated in something a little off the beaten path. For me and for the rest of the participants, it was a healing ceremony, led by a combination of spiritual leaders and medical professionals. Each of us were coming with similar hopes, intentions, and purposes for emotional healing. At the beginning, we sat in a circle, taking time to introduce ourselves and share aloud what we hoped to get out of the time together. Seemingly out of the blue, I felt called to ask for healing for all the unhealed traumas and wounds of my ancestors. I know this probably sounds strange to you, but to be honest, when the impression came over me, I felt a curious, nervous excitement about it.

Reflecting back, it makes a lot more sense now, especially as I continue my journey in recovery. As a therapist and a spiritual coach, I have learned so much about how our genes and environment interact with one another, and how such interactions impact our lives. I sometimes chuckle as I remember our smart-ass remarks when someone was getting on our nerves, and we'd say, "It must be in the DNA." We were half joking, but funny enough, there's actually some solid science behind that Research in genetics and epigenetics suggests that trauma doesn't just affect the person who goes through it—it can literally change how their DNA is expressed, and these changes are passed on to subsequent generations. In other words, the way someone's brain and body respond to stress might be shaped by the experiences of their parents, grandparents, or even further back. It's like a ripple effect through generations. So if someone feels anxious or weighed down by a sense of dread for no obvious reason, it might actually be tied to trauma their family went through long ago.

While the type of spiritual ceremony I'm describing might not seem like something that could actually change a person's brain or biology, there is evidence suggesting it is possible. Just as trauma can influence neurological development and functionality, alongside the expression of our DNA, significant emotional healing can create long-lasting physiological changes in a similar manner. Our bodies are such an amazing, mysterious miracle, aren't they?

In this ceremony, we were led in a style of deep, rapid breathing—which felt intense at first, but after a while, I found myself settling into the flow of it. For those who chose to, there was also the option to drink a tea containing a low dose of psychedelic mushroom "plant medicine." Combining the breathwork with the tea provided the opportunity for deep healing work within a non-ordinary state of consciousness.

I know there's a lot of controversy around the use of plant medicines—especially psychedelics—for medical, mental, or spiritual purposes. While they have been used by indigenous cultures for centuries and were even commonplace in ancient traditions, they also carry the potential for misuse and harm. When you and I talked about it before, I know you had concerns, so trust me when I say, I'm not trying to change your mind or convince you of anything.

All I will say is that there's some compelling research being done by respected institutions like UCLA, Yale, Johns Hopkins, and the National Institutes of Health, with some promising outcomes supporting the clinical use of psychedelics. There is already evidence showing positive changes in neural structure and connectivity that could help individuals overcome trauma, depression, and substance use disorders. Research on ketamine, psilocybin, ibogaine, and ayahuasca has even shown beneficial effects on dopamine and serotonin receptors—the very receptors most often disrupted in those struggling with addiction. That said, the research is still in early stages. I respect that full medical endorsement will require more time and data, so we'll have to wait and see how it unfolds. To me, it is a hopeful potential treatment for the future.

At the same time, I definitely wouldn't encourage someone struggling with addiction to just run out and try mushrooms on their own, hoping for a miracle cure or chasing a new kind of high. I strongly believe that working with this kind of plant medicine requires a safe, supportive setting, skilled facilitation during the experience, and thoughtful integration afterward.

At any rate, let me finish telling you about my experience. In that altered state, I saw myself laying on my back on something like a large altar. Then I saw a long line forming with hundreds of my ancestors, of various ethnicities and sizes, which I took to represent not only biological ancestors from this lifetime, but even ancestors from other lifetimes, if that is a thing.

Each ancestor carried something in their hands, holding it out in front of them—much like the depictions of the wise men in a Christmas nativity scene. But instead of gold, frankincense, and myrrh, I understood that each person was carrying their pains, sorrows, traumas, and grief. I then saw that my whole abdomen had become a large pit, burning hot with fire.

One by one, each ancestor approached me and released their burdens into the fire, where they burned, melted, and disintegrated. I felt the suffering of each of their excruciating pains as they entered the fire within me. I won't lie, this part felt really intense. There was such a deep grief that it felt like someone was emotionally stabbing my heart. As I experienced their anger at the injustices they suffered, my jaw locked, my head throbbed, and my stomach tightened. I felt a paralyzing fear that literally made it hard for me to breathe. At the same time, after each person put their burdens into the fire, they walked away in a manner that appeared so light and free, with dancing, laughter, and peace.

In the end, it was the most incredible healing experience. I felt their pain when they dropped each burden into the fire, but then I felt their freedom and joy once it was burned. What has been even more powerful is that I have continued to feel the positive lasting effects of this healing experience ever since. I feel freer and lighter, like I truly unloaded so much heavy weight. I don't have a before-and-after snapshot of my DNA, but I know something changed. Some sort of deep healing took place, and I really feel the results.

As you and I have talked about so often, our human experience has many layers, and so does the process of healing. When we have opportunities to heal and release the emotional burdens of our past experiences, I believe it brings us to a new level of mental wellness.

I miss you, and as always, am sending my love.

- *L*

14. Runaway Car

"I'll drink to that!" Oh my goodness, how many times did we say that together? Everything was an excuse to drink. While some of those adventures started out fun, many ended "less fun"—or even pretty badly. The truth is that for alcoholics and nonalcoholics alike, everybody initially drinks for the same reasons, at least before the disease takes control. Drinking is not just accepted, it is actually *expected* in so many situations: when we're celebrating at a wedding or party, when we just want to relax, when we've had a bad day, when we're in the midst of stressors or losses…We drink to escape pain, and that's become culturally normal. Have you ever tried counting how many times alcohol shows up on the TV or in a movie? It's almost impossible to watch for an hour without seeing drinking depicted.

What I didn't understand, until doing some reading after rehab, is that for those of us with a biological and neurological predisposition for alcoholism, we just don't have the same "off" switch as "normal" people have. Our brains don't have the same ability to make rational decisions (even when taking a break from drinking), especially after we've been drinking regularly over a period of time. I've been learning that in the brain of a predisposed person who ends up drinking (usually for a variety of "acceptable" reasons), actual physical changes take place that affect long-term decision-making functionality.

It's weird, but I still find myself feeling defensive when people suggest sufferers of a substance use disorder only use because they want the dopamine high. In reality, areas of our brains are literally wired differently. Yes, I know you have jokingly accused me of having something "off," but science is helping me understand better how you may have actually been right. It seems for many of us, the dopamine reward system is, in a sense, "broken." (And that system isn't just about experiencing a high—it is central to the drive and motivation behind most of our decisions.) Add to this the fact that the prefrontal cortex of the brain—the part that controls reasoning and problem solving—is also compromised, causing impaired functioning, even when an addict is sober. So, our motivation system and our rational problem-solving system are both impaired. I love how the authors describe it in their book, *Understanding Addiction—Know Science,*

No Stigma; they say it's like being in a fast-moving vehicle where the brakes aren't working and the steering is out. Can you relate?

This book has a lot of great information on the science and physiology behind substance use disorders, which I wish more people understood. As you know too well, there is such a terrible stigma around addiction, as if it were just a moral issue or personality weakness. We've all heard the accusation that excessive drinking is a "crutch."

Truth is, when you are in the driver's seat of that out-of-control vehicle, it isn't a crutch. If you are speeding down the highway and both your steering and brakes are out, it feels like you literally need a drink to gain control. It feels like basic survival. That isn't true, of course, but the problem with *deception* is that it *deceives* you. Making a rational choice, like not drinking or using, can be almost impossible when your brain is so impacted.

Although it's hard to believe when you feel like you're careening down the highway with no brakes, I'm learning there *is* good news! This brain impairment - both the predisposition and damage after chronic use - doesn't have to be permanent. Even in the depth of disease, even when I couldn't make the choices I needed to about my drinking, I was able to make the choice to let others help me. When I felt helpless and out of control, I called for help, and I was pulled from the car!

These days, I'm just as content sipping a cold, alcohol-free ginger beer or fresh-squeezed lemonade while soaking up the sun on my porch. The drink may be different, but it's still something refreshing I can enjoy with good company. I can sit on that same front porch, in the chairs you know well, and laugh or share stories about the day. Friendships are powerful that way, which brings me to again missing you. Still, I have other special people joining in the laughter and lifting up of spirits - only now without the alcohol or the harm that came with it.

As always, sending my love...

- *L*

15. *Healing My Brain*

Tonight, I'm writing to you while I let my hair dry. I had to wash it after another neurofeedback and neurostimulation session at my daughter's neurotherapy clinic.

"Neuro-what-now," you ask?

These are types of targeted brain treatments that help alter brainwave activity toward healthier patterns of functioning. I'll explain as best I can—but full disclosure, I'm mostly repeating what my provider told me. Writing it out helps me remember, and I think you'll be impressed with my borrowed intelligence.

The process began with a comprehensive QEEG (Quantitative Electroencephalography) brain assessment and an swLORETA 3-D functional analysis. These tests mapped fifty-two different regions of my brain, showing how well (or how poorly) they were functioning and communicating with one another. Basically, the results gave us a roadmap of which areas were healthy, which were struggling, and where things were out of balance.

As I mentioned in my last letter, years of drinking had left a mark on my brain—damage I hadn't even recognized as *brain damage*. My prefrontal cortex (the part responsible for rational thinking, decision-making, and impulse control) was underpowered and struggling to do its job. Meanwhile, my limbic system (the network that processes emotion and activates the fight-or-flight response) was in overdrive, stuck in a state of heightened stress and reactivity. Other areas of the brain were also dysregulated, but these were the most problematic ones.

It still amazes me that this kind of impairment isn't more commonly acknowledged as a brain injury. Again, you might joke that you *knew* something wasn't right (and I wouldn't blame you!), but to the outside world, I looked mostly the same. I could function in day-to-day life, appearing relatively "normal." It was my decision-making, focus, problem-solving, and emotional reactions that gave me away. People didn't see my irrational choices as the result of a compromised brain; they just saw *me*

59

being unreasonable. And while that was partly true, it wasn't the *whole* story.

That's where neurofeedback and neurostimulation came in. These treatments didn't just help repair the damage—I was shocked to learn they also reduced cravings (more like desperate urgings) for the alcohol. They allowed me to make better choices, stabilize my emotions, and maintain my sobriety in those crucial early months. The therapy also calmed my nervous system and supported my trauma recovery, reducing the triggers that would have otherwise sent me reaching for a drink to numb out.

Without this kind of targeted brain intervention, it likely would've taken years for my brain to return to healthy functioning. No wonder relapse rates are so high in the first year of sobriety—people are trying to rebuild their lives while their brain is still working against them.

When I had my first brain scan shortly after my thirty-day rehab stay, my results were a mess—a *dangerous* mess. But after a month of nearly daily targeted neurotherapy, my post assessment showed my brain was "mostly" functioning within normal limits. And more important - I actually *felt* normal again. Or, you know, as normal as I'll ever be (haha!).

There aren't words to describe how grateful I am to have had access to this treatment. It's available to most people, yet it's still relatively unknown and rarely covered by insurance. Now that I understand how powerful it is, it would be a *no-brainer* (yes, lame pun intended) to do it all over again.

I still do occasional neurofeedback and neurostimulation sessions to maintain, improve, and optimize my brain function. It feels like I've been given a fresh start—a new and improved motherboard, so to speak. The only downside? Having to wash the goopy gel out of my hair after each session. But I'd say that's a small price to pay for getting my brain back.

All that said, thinking more clearly doesn't help me miss you less. Know I'm sending my thoughts and love your way.

- *L*

16. *When Did You Stop Dancing?*

Listening to an oldie but goodie right now. Remember the Bee Gees' "You Make Me Feel Like Dancing?" I can't help but smile as I picture you and me singing it together, moving our bodies like no one was watching. I've always loved to dance, though I have to admit it's been a while.

My husband and I used to dance a lot in our dating days and early marriage. We were fearless about it, too. I'll never forget doing the polka in my big, fancy wedding dress, swirling and spinning, taking up the whole room. We even made up our own silly dances—our infamous "happy feet dance" is still a family classic. It's the kind of thing our kids and grandkids love to tease us about to this day. I laugh when I think about us in the early eighties taking a ballroom disco class. Can you imagine it? Swinging to the Bee Gees or Elton John, polyester and all?

However, in the early years of our marriage, there were also a lot of "missteps," not so much in dancing, but in everything else. It seemed like life continued to bring one challenge or disappointment after another, and we eventually stopped dancing altogether. The rhythm of life was lost, and the music seemed to fade away. Somewhere along the way, I think my heart gave up the desire —even the hope—of finding joy in dance again.

I hadn't really thought about how or why that happened until I went to rehab and met a counselor called "Spiritual Steve." One day, he paused, looked each of us in the eye, and asked, "When did you stop dancing?" He asked this before knowing anything about our stories, and before *we* knew anything about what to expect in the group. He went on to explain that his inquiry came from a set of four traditional questions that shamans tend to ask those seeking help for emotional or physical illness:

- When did you stop dancing?
- When did you stop singing?
- When did you stop feeling enchanted by stories?
- When did you become uncomfortable with the sacred territories of silence?

These questions felt like a sudden freezing rain, numbing my mind and body as I felt waves of shock piercing through me. I realized I had lost all the joy and pleasure of living. From the look on the faces around the room, I was in good company. The counselor then prompted us to write our personal stories of what led to the absence of these four things.

Wow. Where do I begin? What led to the fragmented, broken pieces of my existence? As you know, it wasn't just one thing in my life. It was several things over time—many small sufferings, and a few really big heartbreaks. I won't lie, it seemed like an overwhelming assignment. However, denying these things had led me to this dark place. If I wanted a different outcome, I needed to do something different. So many things felt like shards of broken glass—pieces that could never be put back together. Then again, I didn't want to simply rebuild the life I was trying to escape.

Did I start with my marriage, which had teetered on the edge of collapse more times than I could count? Or the financial stress that had loomed over us like a storm cloud, making every decision feel like a desperate juggling act? Then there were my health issues—Crohn's disease, relentless back pain, blood clots, spinal infections, precancerous cells on my ovaries—all of these leading to major surgeries. With all the pain meds, the sleep aids, and my completely out-of-whack hormones, the feeling of sobriety had already slipped away—long before the alcohol took center stage.

I suppose I should acknowledge the heart wrenching deaths in my family—tragedies that left lasting scars. Losing my father was hard enough. But losing a young grandchild to such a brutal illness made me question the very nature of God. That grief not only broke my heart—it shattered my faith. And in many ways, that may have been the most painful loss of all.

As my drinking increased, so did the strain in my relationships with my now-grown children. Becoming estranged from the kids I had always felt so close to shook my world like a violent earthquake—nothing felt stable or secure. I hoped and prayed all would not be lost, but there were times I wasn't so sure.

There were years of insane stress and unreasonable pressures in my job, when no matter what I gave, it was met with criticism. I chose the field of mental health because I wanted to help people. I have genuinely enjoyed being a caregiver in a variety of roles, but over time, the flame I once used to warm others began to burn me up. I was worn so thin that the energy in my heart felt like the fading light at dusk.

So there I was—ready (or not) to bear my soul. While I did the best I could during my time in rehab, much of my healing journey has unfolded (and continues to unfold) in the years that followed. You see, the last step in Steve's exercise was to extend love, forgiveness, and compassion to all these wounded parts of myself. To find acceptance, with grace and understanding, allowing these fragmented parts to heal so they can reunite in the best possible way for health and wholeness.

This last piece was the hardest, because it involved moving out of my ego state of fear and defensiveness, which some part of me believed was keeping me safe, even when it was quite destructive. I hadn't really put this together until Steve called us out on it. In fact, there's another practice he taught us that I can totally imagine you doing with gusto. Before we entered the group room, he would have each of us reach up and slap the doorframe to symbolize "leaving the ego outside." He explained it is the ego that holds on to shame and fear, preventing us from receiving deeper healing. When we can show up with an open and willing heart, leaving our ego "outside," we create space to reconnect with the joys and wonders of life again.

I find myself returning to these teachings time and again, amazed at how far I've come since that day in rehab. Perhaps the practice of consciously setting aside my ego, embracing self-compassion, and approaching life with renewed openness has truly shifted something inside. Today, as I reflect on the four questions, the bitter chill has melted away, replaced by a gentle, glowing warmth. I feel a free and joyful "lightness." Who would have believed so much could change in such a short time, especially after so many years of being miserable? I cherish the sacredness of silence. I love hearing and engaging in stories—even writing them. I sing regularly, whether in the car or in harmony with others. And, at last, my heart is dancing once again.

In fact, more than just my heart is dancing again. Last night at a friend's wedding, my husband and I hit the dance floor with our favorite swing and signature moves, just letting loose and having fun. As we were leaving, we overheard a young couple telling our daughter, "It was so cute watching your parents dance!" Yes, I guess we are now that cute old couple on the dance floor! And I hope we keep dancing for many years to come.

Missing you and sending my love...

- *L*

17. *The Four Agreements*

I didn't know I was so disagreeable! Okay, well maybe *you* knew, and I thank you for loving me anyway. That's what friends are for, right? But it took reading Don Miguel Ruiz's *The Four Agreements* to truly see it for myself. What a powerful book. It was recommended in my IOP (intensive outpatient program) group, but I honestly think anyone could benefit from the ancient Toltec wisdom passed down through its pages. And right now, I hope you'll allow me to practice what I have learned with you. I really want to let it sink in.

The first agreement: **Be impeccable with your word.**

Ruiz says that our words have the power to create or destroy. They can bring beauty and healing—or leave damage in their wake. As you know, I've been quite talented at both. I have spoken words that lifted people up and words that cut people down. I've told truths that mattered and lies that kept me hidden. I know I'm not alone in this struggle.

Being impeccable with our word means choosing integrity. It starts with the thoughts we allow and flows into the way we speak. Just the other day, someone asked why I was late to a meeting. A part of me wanted to offer a "socially acceptable" excuse instead of the truth. But dishonesty, no matter how small, only leads to disconnection. When I present falsely, I rob others of the chance to know and accept the *real* me. Instead of deepening relationships, I create distance. Instead of trust, I build doubt.

So, I'm working on being mindful before I speak—asking myself: is it honest? Is it kind? Is it necessary? Will these words create something beautiful? I think about how I use my words with my granddaughter when I teach her piano—gentle, patient, encouraging. And I contrast that with the cutting words I once hurled in anger at my family when I was drinking words fueled by defensiveness and falsehoods, leaving a wake of damage. It's humbling to admit.

I know I'm still repairing relationships, but I also know that choosing my words carefully now will help build something new—something real and beautiful.

The second agreement: **Don't take anything personally.**

This one has been *hard* for me. I have spent so much energy feeling personally wounded even by total strangers—rude drivers, full sign-up lists, job rejections, restaurant servers who were having an off day. Especially in years past, every little slight carried the threat of a personal attack, as if the universe had singled me out.

And when I was drinking, that defensiveness was multiplied. Whether it was irrational thinking, heightened emotions, or the cloak of shame, I reacted as if everything was *about me*. Someone's in a bad mood? Clearly, it was my fault. A missed invitation? Proof of rejection. I became fluent in verbal aggression, passive aggression, and emotional withdrawal—none of which ever brought me peace.

Today, I understand everyone is on their own journey, carrying their own burdens. People's words and actions reflect their own inner world, not necessarily mine. Even if someone's anger is directed at me, it's still about *them*—where they are in that moment, what they are struggling with, what they need to heal.

And here's where grace comes in. We are all just trying to figure out this thing called life, stumbling through its complexities. Instead of assuming the worst, I want to meet people with understanding. And if I find myself feeling defensive, I want to pause and remind myself: *This isn't about me.* Sure, I want to pay attention to the part of me that is reacting, that needs healing, but I want to let the rest go.

The third agreement: **Don't make assumptions.**

Oh, stop rolling your eyes—I *am* improving! You and I both know I've been guilty of jumping to conclusions, sometimes *leaping* to them. And not just assuming—I often believed I *knew* better than others. Remember our old joke? "People who think they know everything are really annoying to those of us who do." Well, I'll say it: In fact, I don't know everything. In the scheme of things, I find myself better off with the attitude of "I know nothing."

Ruiz describes assumptions as a form of emotional poison. They lead to misunderstandings, unnecessary conflicts, and even wars. I think about all the times I assumed someone's silence meant disinterest, or a delayed response meant rejection. Like when you promised to call me "first thing in the morning," and I was upset when you didn't ring until 11 a.m. I had assumed "first thing" meant 8 a.m., but you had never actually said that.

Assumptions easily morph into expectations, and expectations set us up for disappointment. Now, instead of filling in the blanks with my own narratives, I'm remembering to ask. I will clarify. And I'm finding that people appreciate the chance to explain themselves. It turns out, most misunderstandings can be unraveled with a simple inquiry.

The fourth agreement: **Always do your best.**

This one ties everything together. We live these agreements not through perfection, but through practice. Day by day, moment by moment, I try to apply what I've learned, just like the Alcoholics Anonymous philosophy of "one day at a time." Some days I fall short. Some days I catch myself mid-misstep. But what matters is that I keep choosing to do my best.

My best means striving for integrity—being mindful of my words and choosing to create rather than destroy. It means resisting the urge to take things personally. Remembering that everyone carries their own struggles. It means letting go of assumptions and instead seeking truth. And most of all, it means approaching myself and others with balance, grace, and compassion.

So, here's to the best of the best. And here's to you, always in my heart.

Sending love,

- *L*

18. Deceived

I can't wait to share with you the wild things I saw today.

Looking out the window this morning, I got super excited when I saw what looked like a wild turkey perched on an old wooden fence just across the driveway. I grabbed my phone to take a picture, and as I zoomed in for the perfect shot, I found myself chuckling. As it turned out, my wild turkey was just a gray pigeon atop a tree stump. Shaking my head, I marveled at how easily I was fooled. I have been deceived many times throughout my life, sometimes by others and sometimes by stories my own mind tells. The problem with deception is that, at the time, you don't know you are being deceived.

My alcohol use was rooted in one big deception. In the moment, I believed it was going to make things better, whether that was by helping me relax, sleep, or think more creatively. When I experienced high levels of stress, I thought a drink would give me peace. When I was overwhelmed with grief, I thought it would provide relief from the pain. When my body was in physical pain, I believed the alcohol would make it go away. When my insomnia was keeping me awake, alcohol seemed like a reasonable solution to take the edge off. If I was feeling nervous or socially awkward, a drink seemed to boost my confidence.

It's not uncommon for people to chase illusive "easy fixes" in search of peace, and you know I was no exception. (I can see you making that fake bewildered face - like, "who me?.") For some people, a drink here and there can provide relief in these ways. For me, however, it was ultimately unhelpful, regardless of what I believed or tried to convince myself of.

The pigeon-on-a-stump truth is this: When I was experiencing anxiety or overwhelming emotions, alcohol made me numb, not relaxed. It wasn't peace-giving, it was avoidant. Drinking didn't help me sleep better, it knocked me out. Maybe I would fall asleep easier, but I wouldn't stay asleep, and whatever sleep I did get wasn't deep or restful. As for alcohol giving me more confidence or creativity in my communication, that too was a lie. The outcome was actually kind of a crap shoot. Sometimes what I said or how I interacted would be fine, kind of like nice background music. Other times, what came out would sound more like a loud, screeching cat saying inappropriate and hurtful things. (You've seen me without a filter and common sense. Not a pretty picture!)

Anyway, the list of deceptions could go on and on. It was only once I acknowledged the deception that I could take steps toward better choices.

This afternoon, though, I saw something real! I was just strolling along the river path, mesmerized by the soothing sound of the water flowing. The golden leaves danced back and forth in a graceful parade as they floated through the sky, coming down from the surrounding trees. In the distance, just to the side of the trail, I saw an animal. At first, I thought it was a regular cow. After all, I was in Montana, and goodness knows there are a lot of cows there. As I got closer, however, the shape of the head seemed to be more like a donkey. As I got a bit closer still, I realized it wasn't a ranch cow or a donkey, but a moose cow. I felt a zap of excitement as I glimpsed this wild animal unusually located here, in the middle of the town. Contrary to the turkey, which was just a deception, this moose was undeniably real. Yet, both required a closer look to discern deception from reality.

Many indigenous tribes believe the moose represents strength, independence, self-esteem, adaptability, and a deep connection to the natural world. As I gazed at the animal, I was reminded that I don't have to be ensnared by the ego's illusions or deceptions, chasing quick fixes to bypass humility. It's okay for me to accept guidance, wisdom, and support from others who have experience, helping me to see and understand truth. With confidence and grace, I can embrace my personal power while walking my path in curiosity. In quiet presence, I can live in harmony with the rhythms of nature, guided by my inner knowing, without needing to have all the answers. These are the things that bring me true peace.

So, here's to seeing through deception and enjoying what's real. And while I *really* miss you, I pray that you too are experiencing peace where you are.

Sending my love,

• *L*

19. The Undertow

I was recently reminiscing about the time we went to Morro Bay and walked and talked for hours on the beach. You know how much I love the ocean. It has always been the setting of my favorite vacations. From as young as I can remember, my family would spend a week or two every summer camping right on the beach in Ensenada, Mexico. And, growing up in Bakersfield, California, my family was only a two-hour drive from great beaches like Avila, Pismo, and San Luis Obispo. Remember how you and I would go to Avila every spring break week in high school? Talk about a party!

My husband and young family even lived on the coast for a short spell, which was wonderful. And when my husband and I moved our little family to Colorado, my parents moved to Santa Barbara, which meant we still got to enjoy the magnificence of the ocean from time to time. In many ways, it feels like the ocean is in my blood. I have always felt the bigness and goodness of God standing in or before its grand waves.

So, imagine my surprise when this lovely body of water tried to kill me! Truth be told, you could probably say it was my own fault. We were at Hermosa beach in Costa Rica. I had been chastised by lifeguards the previous day, telling me the water wasn't safe this time of year as the changing seasons created a dangerous undertow. But today, the water seemed calmer, and after all, I was a California girl who grew up swimming in the ocean. In my mind, I was still a young, strong swimmer. Never mind that, on this particular day, I was actually in my sixties.

So, you know me, I went on out. I was so brazen that I even told my husband he didn't need to come or worry about me. I had already had one successful swim that morning, though my husband had expressed concern that the current kept taking me way down the beach. Still, I brushed away the worries.

I had swum out past the wave break for a relaxing float on my back that afternoon. The ocean was much warmer than California waters, and I felt happy and at peace…for a while.

At some point, the water started getting choppier. The playful waves grew and taunted me with threats. It was clearly time to swim back to shore. At first, I swam fairly casually, with effort, but without fear. However, my strokes weren't getting me any closer to the shore, and the waves continued to grow into giant dark monsters around me, seeming to gang up and beat me down. I then swam frantically, with all my strength, in between wave breaks, pausing only to duck under the big waves as they crashed over me. With smaller waves, I would have body surfed to the beach, but these waves were big and angry, and my fear of being crushed by them was greater than my fear of drowning.

I kept swimming harder and more intently, but couldn't make any progress. The waves continued to grow and became increasingly erratic. I scanned the beach, looking up and down the shore for anyone to help me. There was literally *no one* on the beach. There had been people sunbathing earlier, but now everything was deserted. There had been lifeguards on the weekend, but it was now Monday, and they were off duty. Why hadn't I trusted their warnings to stay out of the waters?

After desperately trying to make progress with my rapid strokes and kicks, mustering all my strength for what seemed like an hour, my physical energy was nearly spent. I was so exhausted that my arms and legs had just barely enough energy to keep my head above the turbulent waters. I could hardly believe it, but, in exhaustion, I accepted it—I was going to drown.

My only concern was that others would not have peace, as they wouldn't really know what happened to me. They might assume I had drowned, but there would probably be no body. We were also in a foreign country. What if they thought I had been kidnapped? Defeated, I eventually focused on my sense of gratitude for the life I had lived and the wonderful blessings of my full family. I was too tired to entertain regrets at this point, it just was what it was. I wasn't just exhausted, I was surrendered.

Then, seemingly out of nowhere, a surfer came up on a wave right behind me. He could have hit me if I didn't wave my hands, which I did frantically. He dodged me and rode the wave all the way into the beach. I scanned for other surfers, knowing one rarely surfs alone. There were none. I prayed the surfer, now standing on the beach, would turn and look my way. He had the surfboard under his arm like he was going to leave.

Please God, let him turn and see me. Again, I waved frantically. He saw me.

With hope rising, I watched him walk into the water with the board above his head, avoiding the choppy waves. He paddled all the way back out to me. He asked if I needed help, and I gratefully said, "Yes!" Through my gasps for air and multiple "thank yous," he told me to hold tight to his board. The conflicting waves challenged our retreat, but we slowly made progress. Relief washed over me as he paddled us toward the beach until I could finally reach the bottom and walk myself out of the water. This surfer angel literally saved my life.

Apparently, Tommy (the surfer) lived right by the beach. He told me that people die every year doing exactly what I did. At that particular time of year, there are undertows going both directions, simultaneously, creating perilous conditions for even the strongest swimmers. He went on to say that only surfers will even consider going into the water this time of year, but often they won't take the risk.

I had been warned by others, but I thought I knew better. I waved off concern, believing my knowledge and experience were more valid than theirs—even though they were the locals in this land. Once again, my stubbornness, strong will, and ego nearly cost me my life. It keeps happening—different day, different circumstances, yet the same old pattern. It all seems harmless on the front end. After all, I have always embraced the small risks that come with adventure, so I thought I knew where to draw the line to stay safe.

Yet again, my mind drifts back to my drinking days. There were so many times people shared their concerns for my safety and well-being. So many times, people would offer guidance about how to get help or get sober. Sometimes I would try their suggestions, but more often than not, it seemed like they just felt like endless hoops to jump through on my way to eventual failure. It's not that I believed my way would work better, just that after so many failed attempts, I didn't think anyone's way would actually work. I needed a miracle—or a few of them. My ego's bluster couldn't begin to match the strength and potential danger of the ocean *or* substance addiction. It seemed to require divine intervention to survive drowning—whether in a bottle or the ocean.

Of course, today I realize there is immense value in heeding the wise advice of others, especially when they possess knowledge and experience that I lack. I know that sounds obvious, but if I'm honest with myself, sometimes I think I know more than I actually do. So far, I've lived to tell about it, but I hope to avoid such unnecessary risks in the future.

I aspire to remain strong and courageous while also embracing humility and receptivity. I'm realizing that being humble and receptive is very different from shame and helplessness. It actually shows incredible strength and courage to trust others and their wisdom, to believe others have good intentions toward me and for me.

I will continue to love the ocean, but now, I have a new respect for it. When it comes to drugs or alcohol, I will recognize them as something to be respected by some and avoided by others. For me, they will never be safe. For me, it is like a double undertow seeking to take me down. I recognize alcohol will not just take me hostage, it will eventually kill me if I give in to it.

Respecting the power of the ocean doesn't mean I live in fear of it—it means I know my limit and act accordingly. The same is true with alcohol. I don't avoid it out of weakness; I avoid it because I know it will always be stronger than me. And that's not shame—that's wisdom.

It would be so wonderful if you were here to enjoy some fun and healthy adventure with me. Not one that would threaten our lives, just one that would be filled with excitement and joy like the many experiences we have had together in the past. For now, as always, I'm sending my love…

- *L*

20. Steps

Well, here I am again, nursing a scraped and swollen knee. I tripped coming up the porch step to our house. Yes, it's been there a long time—since we bought the house nine years ago, in fact—and yet I still misjudged it and went down. I'm glad it wasn't more serious, but it was enough to make me pause, which led to reflection. As I'm sure you know, this isn't the only step that's tripped me up a little in my life.

We always hear about the twelve steps in AA or similar programs for sobriety. However, I have come to believe there are many more than just twelve. Healing isn't a one-way staircase with twelve neat, linear steps and a metal platform at the top. It's more like a long spiral staircase with all kinds of unexpected obstacles—and sometimes incredible discoveries. I used to think I would climb each step just once and move on, but in reality, I find myself circling the same challenges the twelve steps present over and over—each time with new awareness, new struggles, and new strength.

For example, I feel like steps one, two, and three, are a part of my *daily* routine, now. Not on a conscious level so much, but rather like a part of my morning meditation and prayer. They are all about acceptance and surrender, allowing the love and power of the Divine to give me strength, wisdom, self-control, and ultimately to keep me safe.

Most of us have heard the serenity prayer, which really is a guidepost for me that I reflect on daily. "God, grant me the serenity to accept the things I cannot change, the courage to change the things I can, and the wisdom to know the difference."

Yet, even with this prayer, it isn't always a peaceful climb. There are so many times I feel flabbergasted as I stumble back down and find myself yearning for a drink. The safety net, for me, is in staying connected to a loving "strength that is greater than my own"—a true lifeline. (That and the support of important people like you and my sponsor.)

Then there are steps four and five, which proved to be particularly challenging for me in the moments when I first took the moral inventory. You know, when I had to honestly reflect on how my drinking and actions harmed others. Who wants to look at all their mistakes and inexcusable behaviors? It was humbling when I finally began admitting them out loud to my sponsor. But the beauty of having a sponsor to confess to was knowing that she wouldn't judge me. She had climbed these same high steps and was always ready to help me.

Before step four, I thought drinking was a way to escape pain. But in reality, I was carrying the pain with me the whole time—dragging it around like an old, overstuffed suitcase. When I finally started unpacking it, piece by piece, (which is what step four requires), admitting everything out loud to my sponsor, I expected to feel exposed. But instead, I actually felt lighter. The weight of my own deception lifted. I had taken out the garbage, all that shame and guilt, and for the first time in a long time, I could breathe.

Steps six, seven, eight, and nine revolve around taking responsibility and allowing God, who I see as the Author of Love, to heal and change us. Then we are able to take the necessary steps to make amends, to whatever extent possible, doing what we can to make things right.

Again, as I began this process, it was more than uncomfortable. In the beginning, my throat clenched, and my chest and shoulders tightened every time I sat down with a loved one to start the conversation. It was about apologizing, not asking for forgiveness, even though that was of course what I sought. It was important to acknowledge and share how sorry I was without any expectation of the other person.

One of the hardest conversations I had was with my daughter. I expected anger, maybe rejection. Instead, she listened. She wasn't ready to forgive, and I had to be okay with that. I had done my part, and in doing so, I freed myself from the weight of unspoken regret.

Like my daughter, there were a handful of people who weren't ready to forgive or say it's all okay now. But everyone seemed to appreciate the effort, and they were sincerely grateful I was sober and taking the steps to stay that way. The forgiveness and acceptance did come. It just took some time—after those who cared about me could believe my sobriety was for real. As hard as step nine was, it was honestly the most healing and freeing.

This is another step I find myself practicing now on a daily basis. If I see that I have hurt someone else, whether intentionally or unintentionally, I apologize for my part and try to find peaceful resolution. Conflict is a true stressor, and life feels so much better with less of it. And as I'm getting to experience, true conflict resolution doesn't come from avoiding the issue. Resolution is the blessing of actually addressing an issue with love and seeking a solution together. As I look back, I think getting to practice this with you in the past is what has given us such a rich friendship.

If the earlier steps are about surviving, these later ones are about thriving. They remind me that healing isn't just about what we let go of—it's about what we build, the love we share, and the light we pass on to others who are still climbing the same steps.

To me, steps ten through twelve are about staying open and connected to the Higher Power, bringing out the highest version of ourselves. I really like these steps, because they encourage me to share my hope and light with other sufferers. This is where I like to hang out, in the feel-good place of being a helper and encourager. Yet, I'm only able to serve here authentically after having worked through and "climbed" the steps that came before.

And I don't mind revisiting all these steps as I continue to ascend, floor by floor, on my spiral staircase. Each new level has a spectacular view— broader than the one before. Life is a healing journey full of these moments of growth and connection if we commit to being present and honest, and if we have the courage just to keep going—one foot in front of the other. I can't think about my healing journey without thinking of you. You have been one of many important friends who supported me, helping me stay sober, with kindness and encouragement. My heart feels warm, and a smile spans my face as I reflect on many of the thoughtful things you have said, as well your brutal accountability when necessary!
I miss you, my friend. If you were here, we'd climb another staircase together—just like we always have. But for now, I keep walking, step-by-step, carrying thoughts of you with me.

Sending love,

- *L*

21. *Wearing My Broken Heart*

Today, I wanted to feel love. My heart felt sad and lonely, so I reached for the beautiful rose quartz heart pendant you gave me—the one that has always reminded me of you. I wanted its warmth against my skin, its quiet assurance that love endures. But as I was putting it on, it slipped from my fingers, hitting the floor with a small, sharp sound. When I picked it up, I noticed the tiny chip, a missing piece. And suddenly, I felt the weight of every chip my own heart has endured over the years.

Everyone experiences disappointment or heartbreak at one point or another. I do believe suffering is part of the life process of growing and healing as a person, but still there have been so many times in my life I literally asked God to give me a break from the "growing pains."

Growing up, my family was quite dysfunctional, as most families are at least part of the time. I'm sure you remember some of the stories I have shared about the borderline abuse and neglect of my childhood. You also know the rocky road my marriage has traveled over the years. I cried on your shoulder when my relationships with my children and their spouses were strained. My soul bears scars from the betrayal of best friends, abandonment of what I thought were "true loves," not to mention the literal deaths of family members, friends, and fur angel pets who I sometimes felt closer to than my human companions. Chip after chip has sheared off this heart. I know your story isn't all that different.

For years, I carried resentment like gravel in my pockets—heavy, cold, always pressing against me. Forgiveness didn't mean pretending the slurry never existed; it meant finally emptying my pockets—setting it down. Letting go doesn't mean saying "it's okay." It means deciding it no longer controls me.

So, I decided I didn't want to hold on to all this pain. I no longer wanted to focus on all the disappointments, abuse, neglect, misunderstandings, etc. Bitterness and resentment weren't going to help me get justice—they were only weapons that would end up wounding me instead.

So, I have decided to embark on the practice of forgiveness. As my mentor would say, just release and let gravity take it away. And, though it's unbelievably hard to admit, the truth is I have just as much to forgive in myself for as I do in others.

Some days, forgiving myself is harder than forgiving anyone else. I can tell myself that I was doing the best I could, that I didn't know any better—but there's still that quiet voice whispering, "but you should have." I've learned that trying to silence that voice doesn't work. The only way to quiet it is to sit with it and to tell it, "Yes, I made mistakes. But I don't have to carry them forever."

I'm also learning that, while it is important to not get caught up in shame, it *is* important to take ownership of my actions. I'm learning to take responsibility for my behaviors during my years of drinking, even if some of the precipitating reasons for my addiction weren't my fault. Sure, there were the biological predispositions and physiological reactions within my body that caused the addictive reactions, but the bottom line is, I still made choices and acted on them. At several points, the choices I made eventually hurt others. It was important for me to own them and apologize, to do what I could to make it right for both the people I harmed and myself.

As you've heard me talk about, the ninth step in AA is the practice of making amends by apologizing and trying to make things right. But what about when that isn't really possible? In some cases, it seems to me, now, that making amends is more an act of grace, forgiveness, and acceptance—believing everyone was doing the best they could with the information, mental health, and skills they had at the time—including myself. Even when I've made really bad decisions, there has been a part of me that had a "good" or "justified" reason for doing it. I truly believe we all do the best we can with what knowledge or experience we have in any given circumstance. I can see this in myself, as well as those who've hurt me. We are all "perfectly in process," just trying to figure things out.

While you know how hard this can be for me, offering grace and release for past mistakes either made toward me or by me is an important act of healing. Doing this allows me to move forward freely. Forgiveness is like the key to freedom, while compassion for myself and others is a healing salve.

The truth is, pain and suffering are going to be a part of our journey. Fighting or resisting them and wallowing in misery is only going to cause more pain. If we can in some way accept them as a part of the human experience—seeing them as something *on* our way, not *in* our way, in the process of becoming the highest version of ourselves—we can stay in the flow of life and eventually move forward.

Authentic spiritual wholeness must be open-ended as we are always on the move and in process. For me, it has been helpful to finally recognize that my suffering or dis-ease is not always a sign of something wrong, but actually evidence of something profoundly *right*. C.S. Lewis suggests our conscience is actually a God-given compass pointing toward the standard of love within us. He also suggests, "Hardships often prepare ordinary people for an extraordinary destiny." Understanding that suffering is a part of life's journey toward becoming *the highest version of myself* helps me embrace my broken pieces and scars.

Maybe, unlike rose quartz, living hearts don't have to stay broken. They bruise, they scar, but they also grow. A gemstone stays chipped forever, but hearts, when given love, can reshape themselves around the cracks. Maybe that's why the heart keeps beating—because it refuses to stay shattered.

So today I wear my broken heart, knowing that every crack tells a story. I also know that both the people who have come and gone, and the ones who are here to stay, are part of the family and community I've been given for this life. The pain, ownership, forgiveness, acceptance—it's all an important part of my story, and I'm beginning to understand that it really is through brokenness that I can be my highest authentic self.

Some people left, but you stayed through so many painful and hard times. You truly are a part of my heart. Because of that, it isn't just chipped—it is also whole.

Sending my love,

- *L*

22. *The Messengers*

A really sad thing happened yesterday, and I need to talk to someone. I'm able to write through some tears tonight, but yesterday I just couldn't stop crying. I sure wish you were here in person, but I guess writing to you will have to suffice.

I was at the dining room table eating lunch alone, and suddenly, there was a loud thud that shook the house. Just as I paused, mouth open for another bite, there was another thud. My stomach clenched. Was someone pounding on the door? I hesitated, my heart already racing as I went to check. As I cautiously opened the front door, my breath caught in my throat. A large, brilliantly colored bird lay motionless on the porch, and a smaller one just like it stood watching me just about three feet away in the flower bed.

Their primary color was such a brilliant bright blue, with white chests and an orangey rust colored belt across their abdomens. I knew these birds from photos—Kingfishers.

My heart ached as I saw the larger adult bird laying on the porch in front of me. At first it looked peaceful lying there, and I hoped it was just in shock. The younger bird—clearly shaken—was waiting, too. I don't know how long I stood there, but eventually, it became clear: the large bird had died on impact.

As I stood there stunned, its brilliant blue feathers seemed to be slowly dimming in the sunlight. The smaller one, trembling a few feet away, began crying out over and over—its voice thin and desperate. It wasn't just calling. It was *pleading*. It didn't understand. It didn't know that no matter how many times it called, the answer it longed for would never come.

I hesitated to move toward the young bird, not wanting to frighten it more. But I thought it must be injured, and I so badly wanted to help. Eventually, when I took a step out from the doorway, the little one flew up in retreat. But as though there was an invisible string tied between this little bird and its parent, it didn't fly far. It took roost on a branch in a nearby tree and continued to cry out.

My own tears started flowing as I witnessed all of this, and I could barely swallow. Just a few months ago, I sat by the bedside of my own mother, watching her as she died. Her face flashed in my mind, and standing there in the doorway, my grief once again began to overtake me.

Did that young bird on the wire understand death? Was it just learning the terrible pain of loss in this moment? Maybe out of my own grief—or maybe to try to help that young Kingfisher understand—I decided to leave the poor thing's parent on the porch for a couple of hours. Still, even at dawn the next morning, long after I had removed its parent from the porch, the young bird was perched on the branch, crying out and waiting. Loss is just so hard.

I guess it doesn't matter what kind of animal you are, death is a part of life and grieving is something we all have to work through at some point.

The weight of this moment felt too significant to ignore. Kingfishers are rare where I live, and two of them appearing like this—one surviving, one not—felt like a message. So, in my search for comfort and meaning, I turned to the stories and folklore surrounding these birds.

First, I learned that kingfisher is another name for halcyon—a word that represents a time in the past that was idyllically happy and peaceful. I let that sit with me for a moment. That's beautiful and all, but this happy little symbol of peace died on my doorstep. The irony of it stung.

It reminded me of the early days of my drinking. In the beginning, alcohol seemed to give me a sense of fun and freedom, a kind of manufactured peace. Until, at some point, without warning, it turned deadly. What had seemed fine—normal, even—became a slow unraveling of everything I thought I could hold together.

I read on. Another source said that when a kingfisher arrives in your life, it signals abundance, courage, and prosperity. That it's a sign of a new chapter. It encouraged me to "open my wings and fly on the winds of opportunity, facing what's ahead, head on."

Umm…that's literally how this bird died.

I sat there, shaking my head, wondering if the universe was just messing with me at this point. But then I saw something else.

Kingfisher spirit is said to show up when you're struggling with fear. It urges you to stop hiding, to stop shrinking back, to push forward toward something greater. And there it was.

Because while I've always been a risk-taker in some ways—skydiving, riding a motorcycle, traveling without plans or safety nets—there's a whole other kind of fear that's always lurking beneath the surface. The fear of putting myself out there and risking failure or rejection.

I've spent years holding back, being afraid to fully step into the things that make me feel alive, like art, music, writing, and being creative. And yet, after becoming sober and making the necessary changes in my life to maintain sobriety, I have found myself at a series of crossroads. I literally get to redefine who I am. I feel things shifting and I have no choice but to move forward.

I looked again at that young bird, still lingering, still processing the loss. I put my hand to my heart and allowed the tears to drip down my face. I still feel the sadness even as I find some new meaning in it. (And I am thankful to God for the comfort that brings today.) All life is sacred. This beautiful bird's life ended, just as my mom's did, while its youngster's and mine continued.

And maybe, that's the most important message.

That even after loss, there is survival.

That even after collision, there is flight.

That grief does not mean the end of everything—it means transformation.

As I searched further, I found another interpretation—one that speaks of renewal, transition, and protection. A reminder that just because something has ended doesn't mean all is lost. And perhaps that's the real meaning of finding a bird on your doorstep.

So, as I sit here, breathing in the stillness of this moment, I realize something. If I were still drinking, I wouldn't have been able to receive messages like this. I wouldn't be present enough to see them, to feel them, to let them shape me. Sobriety has given me a kind of clarity I never had before. It has given me the ability to stand at a crossroads and not be paralyzed by fear. To not run, to not numb, and to trust.

Before the sun set yesterday, I laid the Kingfisher into the earth. Death is never an end—it is a return. A return to the soil, to spirit, to the great unknown. And yet, even as I whisper this truth to myself, my heart still aches. I still want to hear my mother's voice, just as that young bird longs for its parent's song.

I like to believe that somewhere, the spirit of that Kingfisher still soars. That my mother, too, is free. And that both of them—somewhere beyond my sight—are at peace.

As Hafiz once wrote:

> Know the true nature of your beloved.
>
> In his loving eyes, hear every thought,
>
> word, and movement as always, always, beautiful.

And so, I listen, I trust, and I keep moving forward.

Sending my love,

- *L*

23. *The Luminous Shadow*

Tonight, the full Hunter's Moon hung in the sky like a lantern against the velvet dark. A silver ring circled it—an omen of coming rain. Yet, as I stood beneath it, the moon felt less like a warning and more like a watchful eye, staring down upon me, steady and luminous. It felt…alive.

Could you see it from where you are?

The beautiful contrast of light and dark brought to mind how we so often think about light as "good" and dark as "bad." The truth is, both are equally important as two ends of a spectrum that is, ultimately, good. They are both parts of the experiences that shape us into who we are.

This brought to mind a conversation I once had with a third-grade girl named Estrella, which means "star" in Spanish. In response to one of my questions, she responded that black was her favorite color. Having expected the usual response—pink, maybe purple—I asked why she chose black. She smiled, her eyes glowing with certainty. "Because," she said, "it's in the black sky that stars shine their brightest."

Her words landed deep, like a forgotten truth suddenly remembered. How had I never thought of it that way? Without the dark, the stars would be invisible—just as, without our struggles, our joys would have nothing to shine against.

"Oh, the wisdom from the mouths of babes," I can hear my mom say.

For the past few years, I've done a lot of what is called *shadow work*—a process of recognizing and healing what seem to be inherent weaknesses or shortcomings, such as fears or beliefs that impact our choices and daily living. For me, this journey has involved acknowledging and working to heal things like the fear of rejection or wanting life to always be joyful and fun. It has also meant facing past traumas, grief that impacts all parts of my being, and the mistakes, weaknesses, and shame I've carried, as these are all parts of my shadow.

You and I have talked about our shadow parts before, particularly when we found ourselves desiring things or acting in ways that weren't in alignment with our higher values. In his book, *On the Brink of Everything*, Parker Palmer describes them as "anything that we can't or won't see about ourselves, or the parts we feel so deeply ashamed of that we hide them." He goes on to say, "We have this amazing capacity for self-deception, so our shadows are often very well hidden. Because of this hiddenness they tend to have power over us. Our shadows are not 'evil'; they just allow us to do harm and not know it."

For so many years, I ran from my shadows. I drank to keep them buried, to silence the voices that relentlessly whispered of my failures, my regrets, my deepest wounds. But the thing about shadows is that ignoring them doesn't make them disappear. They only grow stronger. They seep into your choices, your relationships, your self-worth. They are no longer just shadows, but puppeteers pulling your strings.

It wasn't until I turned to face them that they lost their power. The light didn't destroy them; it transformed them.

When we address our pains, challenges, false beliefs, and negative behaviors, we allow these shadow parts to heal and integrate into our whole being. I have finally come to a place where I can better embrace the shadows in my life and see them as an important part of my soul journey. In gaining understanding of them, I have become a stronger and better person.

While I am grateful for the lessons of shadow work, I understand it is not a "one and done" event. It is a daily process of acknowledging and releasing what is not helpful for my highest good. That is the only way healing can continue. There is an exercise I've done regularly with my clients over the years that involves writing out every mean or abusive thing someone else has done to cause pain, fear, anger, or deep sadness.

Every time I do this exercise with a client, it takes me back to the first time I did this ritual for myself at the beginning of my healing journey in sobriety. After writing out absolutely everything I could think of that caused me suffering, anger, or despair, I placed the pages in a small metal trash bin. I struck the match and lit the paper. As the flames curled around the paper, I watched the words blacken and shrivel, then crumble into ash. The stories of hurt, of loss, of old wounds long carried—they dissolved into smoke, rising like whispers to the night sky. The fire didn't erase them, but it changed them. And in doing so, it changed me.

The residual pain, trauma, grief, and brokenness don't actually leave us, but they can change form into something helpful for our personal development. When I think of the most beautiful, loving, and good people I know, I reflect on all the grief or tragedy they've experienced in their lives. It's always a part of their story. When one allows healing in these deep, broken-heart parts, a beautiful transformation takes place. From the healed shadow, one attains great compassion and understanding. This, in turn, provides opportunities for substantial spiritual growth and guidance in our life purpose.

Just as Yin is to Yang, I see that my difficult and traumatic experiences— including my poor choices and consequences—are just as important and valuable to my overall life as the "light" experiences. Yet, the shadow side is only helpful when we utilize it as a growth platform. As I reflect on the shadow work I have done, I see that by addressing and healing the dark side or painful issues in my life experience, I have become a more positive, supportive, and loving person. An "estrella" in the dark of a seemingly black night.

Goodnight for now, my dear friend. Wherever you are, I hope you can see the same moon shining above you, a quiet promise in the dark. If the stars need the dark to shine, maybe we, too, need our shadows to become whole. Maybe healing is simply learning to reflect the light we've always carried within us—like the moon reflecting the sun, even in the blackest sky.

As always, sending my love…

- *L*

24. *Whispers in the Wind*

"It's a blustery day" as Winnie the Pooh would say—a day when the wind doesn't just drift by but rushes in, playful and wild. The trees surrender their golden leaves, sending them swirling like tiny dancers to an otherworldly waltz. Even the ground isn't still. A golden carpet ripples as if the earth itself is breathing.

You know how I've always loved the wind. It used to annoy you, if I remember correctly. In fact, I believe most people don't like it very much. But I love it. I feel hope and renewal as it blows against my face, caressing me with a cool burst of freshness. It doesn't bother me if it messes my hair or ruffles my clothes. When I was younger, I remember dancing in the wind, even in the sprinkles of rain, delighted in the interaction with the elements.

To me, wind is always ushering in some sort of change. Some people fear change, resist it, but I've often sought ways to create it. Every few months, I'd rearrange furniture, repaint walls, or reinvent some small part of my world. Maybe I was searching for a feeling, a reminder that life is never stagnant, that we aren't stuck.

And yet, there have been plenty of changes I didn't choose—of the kind that steals the breath from your lungs. The kind that comes like a storm and leaves you wondering who you are now. Those…I haven't been so eager to embrace. But the wind doesn't ask for permission. It moves, it shifts, it carries. And maybe that's what hope is—trusting that the wind knows where it's going, even when we don't.

When I watch wind in nature, I feel this sense of excitement and hope, because I know that seeds are blowing and planting and bedding themselves deep into the earth to create new life. I have this belief that something good is coming.

I think there's such a great and important power in hope. In fact, that is the main reason I decided to pursue counseling as a career—I wanted to help people find hope. I aspired to be the kind of messenger of hope that Parker Palmer describes: "A messenger who really has nothing to do with cheering others on, but rather one who enters into relationships that honor the soul, encourage the heart, inspire the mind, and helps to heal the wounds we suffer along the way." Having known people who have ended their lives and worked with so many people who have lost loved ones to suicide, I know the consequences and pain for all involved when there is such a deep loss of hope.

You can imagine the contrast and even desperation I felt when I, a therapist, was deep in my own addiction and not even feeling hope for myself. When one is without hope, the world is so dark. It's hard to breathe. You know the feeling, don't you? When you wake up and realize, once again, nothing has changed. The tunnel is just as dark, the walls just as suffocating. And so, you drink—to quiet the thoughts, to soften the edges. But the relief is temporary, and when it fades, somehow the tunnel has grown even longer, the walls even closer.

Hopelessness isn't just a feeling—it's a weight, a heaviness that, when carried long enough, you forget what it's like to walk without it.

Hope is not overrated. It's easy to hope for some things that are very likely to happen, like anticipating a party that you hope will turn out well. There are other times when hope is harder—like when we hope that someone we love can overcome a terrible illness, despite their prognosis. For those suffering in the throes of addiction, when we can muster it, the hope is that life will someday be worth living again. As you know all too well, it really is that dark…at least it was for me.

When I finally submitted to going into treatment for the second time, I can't say I believed it would work. After all, I had gone through detox before—yes, without the full rehab program—but still, within two months, I was drinking again. There are no words to describe the intense feeling of failure and hopelessness I felt at that point. The money we had to pay out of pocket, down the drain. The pity and frustration those around me expressed at my defeat was like an ominous shadow looming over me. Those were the days I could barely function, spending day after day in bed, literally avoiding eye contact with anyone, as my shame seemed to swallow me whole. I didn't go to work. I barely ate. And of course, I drank.

So, if you had asked me whether I thought sobriety would actually stick after another stint in rehab, I wouldn't have even given it a fifty-fifty chance. I had read the statistics about how few people are successful at overcoming this disease. I didn't feel stronger or more special than anyone else. I honestly didn't know if I could even do it again. This time committing to the full program (which also meant putting out a lot more money), I could only hope—against all my doubts—that it would somehow work. That I would be able to stay sober. That kind of hope might sound simple, but I guarantee you it wasn't easy. It would have been nice to know then what I know now about all the important practices and treatments of a good rehabilitation program. I had done a little research before I went in, but mostly, I lucked out. My program ended up being one of those in the one percent that use all the evidence-based medications, quality medical care, and support of licensed mental health staff, with interventions focused on not just the physical and emotional, but also the spiritual wellness of the patients. As I've mentioned before, I think it's in this spiritual component that hope either flourishes or it doesn't.

That's why I love the wind—it reminds me of the unseen forces at work in our lives. I may not always know where it's taking me, but I trust that something greater does. Whether we call it God, the creator, mother earth, or simply love, I believe in a force that moves us forward, even when we feel stuck.

For me, spiritual hope comes through a multitude of representations and strengths. First and foremost, I believe in God, a traditional higher power. But I also joyfully connect and find support through many of the bazillion other beautiful options that represent the paragon of love and goodness. I personally don't think the source of divine love cares by what name you connect—only that you do, so that it can be that lifeline, that source of hope we all need on a daily basis.

I understand some changes won't be comfortable or pleasant. I know some seeds won't grow into new life. Still, I have a peace and an excitement in the process—in the core belief that, at some level, every season is good and important. While I might not enjoy winter as much as I enjoy spring or summer, I know it's an important part of the process.

That being said, I think I'll sign off and step outside. The wind is calling, carrying its unseen magic, and I want to feel it on my skin—to let it remind me that I am alive, that change is constant, and that hope is always, always in motion. I imagine you here with me—standing in the gusts, arms open, letting the wind pick up what no longer serves us and carry it far, far away. The changes and transformations are taking root, with hope, all will be well.

As always, sending my love...

- *L*

25. *Holding Loosely*

Today, grief lingers like a shadow. I woke up missing my mom, missing you, missing so many who have either moved away or passed on. Some days, the weight of loss feels heavier than others, as if my heart is sifting through memories, reluctant to let them fade. I feel like I've already lost so much in this lifetime. And yet, life keeps asking me to let go of more.

The older I get, the more I realize that so much about life is learning how to let go. My mother would often say, "Growing old is a gift." This was usually mentioned in the wake of learning a friend had passed away, or when enduring a new loss.

Even in childhood, loss is woven into the rhythm of life. We outgrow our favorite shoes, leave behind beloved teachers, watch friendships shift like the seasons. We shed pieces of our innocence, often before we're ready. No one prepares us for the fact that growing up comes with a series of goodbyes.

Some loss is a natural part of the growth process, while others are a result of our choices and behaviors. Anyone who has experienced substance addiction will tell you stories of all the great losses that come with the disease. Many lose their families, marriages, jobs, homes, health, or even freedom. Many people have to start over with new jobs or careers, as well as new friend groups as they change to hanging with a sober crowd.

Through my behaviors while in my addiction, I lost so much more than just external things. I was fortunate to not lose all the things I just mentioned, but the things I did lose, at least temporarily, were of great importance. I lost any resemblance of self-respect, self-confidence, and sense of self-worth. I lost many friendships and, for those who hung in there with me, I lost the comfort and ease that goes along with positive communication, safety, and trust. Anger and frustration were constant, unwelcome guests, compromising the comfort or joy in any regular companionship. All relationships were strained.

With loss comes grief. Grief can be devastating and lonely. It can leave us feeling adrift and confused in the middle of life, or at least that is how it was for me.

However, just like the rainbow and sun appearing after a terrible storm, the loss felt around my addiction transformed into something more like a new birth. There was a new beginning and opportunity to redefine myself. In starting over, I was able to rebuild my value and belief structure. I was able to develop relationships from a new and healthier place of authenticity. In my work, I was able to better serve my clients from a place of wholeness and acquired wisdom.

There were numerous smaller losses as well—ones that may not have led to great changes in identity, but still became catalysts of new transitions and positive movement. While I admit, it was sometimes really hard to release my hold on certain things I thought I needed, I found freedom in letting go.

I think the hardest part of all the loss around addiction is the shame I've felt over the thought that it could have all been avoided. Shame whispers in my ear late at night, looping the same cruel stories: "You should have known better. You wasted too much time. You hurt the people you love."

There are so many *if onlys*. If only I had never started drinking at all. If only I had gone into treatment sooner. If only I had understood then what I know now. Of course, *if onlys* don't have any benefit and they certainly don't bring peace, but I think they were a natural part of my sobriety process.

It's an unforgiving script, and it took me a long time to realize something: regret and shame are not the same thing. Regret acknowledges the past; shame chains you to it. If I was ever going to heal, I had to loosen my grip on both.

I used to think holding on was a sign of strength, but the longer I live, the more I see that there is strength in knowing when to release. Not with bitterness, not with resistance, but with trust that life is still unfolding in good ways we can't yet understand.

Truth is, in getting sober, pretty much everything changed. In fact, most of the things that had become familiar and commonplace in my world *had* to be different. I "lost" alcohol as a coping strategy, which forced me to develop new skills and practices—which was such a good thing! I was forced to redefine myself, which led to the changes in me I always wanted to make.

Letting go of the inaccurate messages we've been told throughout our lives seems to be part of everyone's journey—not just those struggling with addiction. Messages of unworthiness or unlovability were merely other people's projections and emotional garbage put upon us. We see this in families all the time—parents projecting their shame upon their children or passing down misguided beliefs that love and worthiness must be earned. You get the picture.

Growing up, most of us believed these projections to be true about ourselves, and the world's expectations seem to further make the point. In my journey, however, once I recognized this damaging, faulty belief system, I had the option of releasing and letting go of the untruths. This created for me the new beginning I just described. It gave me an opportunity to live out of my highest values, knowing I am lovable and worthy and valuable simply because I exist.

This was actually quite an uncomfortable part of my healing process. It felt scary, like I was losing a part of myself, my identity, as I shed those lies. In reality, it was like I was taking off a costume that I had mistakenly believed was my identity. The deception of alcohol had been like looking in the funny mirror at a circus, distorting all reality, to the point I didn't even know who I was anymore. So, losing that false and confused image was a blessing, and starting from scratch to recreate the me I wanted to be was a gift. While these losses may not have felt like good things when they were happening, the end result has been better than I could have imagined.

I like how John O' Donohue puts it, "Loss always has much to teach us; its voice whispers that the shelter just lost was too small for our new souls."

What I have come to realize is that some loss is not only good for us, but necessary. Yes, my transformation through healing started by letting go of the alcohol. This was a necessary first step, but thankfully there was even more loss. You see, becoming our most authentic selves happens as we let go—piece by piece—of the old definitions, old identities, old belief systems that keep us small or limited. It's undoing all that the world puts on us—all the gunk that, over time, obscures our pure, divine core. I believe it is at this core that we are most like God.

If indeed we are made in the image of God (as several religions and spiritual practices claim), we can believe we are, in essence, perfect, with inherent worth and divine purpose. This is who we are in our most authentic, beautiful self. So, if I have to lose, let go, wash off a bunch of trash, slime, and lies to get to that divine authentic core, I embrace that loss.
Some losses we make peace with. Others leave an emptiness we simply learn to carry.

Losing alcohol was a gift. Losing the false versions of myself was freedom. But losing people we love? That's a different kind of loss that just doesn't feel right. Be that as it may, know that I am sending you my love and hugging you with my heart. The friendship we share is an everlasting one—no matter the distance, we'll always stay connected.

Sending my love,

- *L*

26. Beauty, Pain, and A Little Bird Poop

So, this just happened. I was heading out to meet some friends for coffee when I noticed a lovely flock of small birds perched in a flowering tree above me. I paused for a moment, taking in their simple beauty, and listening to their sweet, lyrical sounds. I even sang a little "good morning" back to them. But when I stepped forward, they startled and took flight, and—you guessed it—one pooped on my head.

I stood there for a second, stunned, and then I laughed. Of course. Life has a way of delivering both beauty and mess in the same breath.

It reminded me of that time in Ensenada when we saw a pelican on the beach. We were excited to see it so close to us, especially when it didn't fly away as we approached. It was clearly injured, crying out, but when you tried to get close enough to help, it lashed out, trying to bite you. We, as people, aren't so different. How often do we strike out in pain, even at those who mean us no harm?

I think about the many meaningful relationships I've been blessed to have over the years. I also think about the wounds that have come with them. Friends I trusted who betrayed me. Loves I believed in who broke my heart. Family who misunderstood and judged me. Jobs I poured myself into that still ended badly. Relationships that just…faded away.

With each hurt, I recoiled a little more. It felt safer to keep people at a distance than to risk another disappointment. What I didn't realize then is that protecting myself from pain also meant closing myself off from joy. I was so focused on what had gone wrong that I couldn't see how everything—even the hard stuff—was shaping me for good.

I see it differently now. Every experience, good or bad, was a valuable part of my life journey. Even the heartbreaks. Even the betrayals. Even the times I felt lost and alone. Each one was an invitation to grow, to understand myself better, to heal the parts of me that needed attention.

Of course, that kind of clarity took time. When I was drinking, my relationships were strained, if not outright broken. I told myself alcohol made things easier, but in reality, it only deepened the distance. I longed for connection, yet I kept pushing people away. I think of the saying we've often reflected upon: "Hurt people hurt people." Sadly, that was my story. I was hurt, and I hurt others, which in turn led to more hurt. It didn't take much to hurt my feelings those days. And I numbed it all. In doing so, I lost the very thing I was aching for—real closeness, real love, real belonging.

Sobriety changed that. Slowly, I began to rebuild—not just my relationships, but my sense of self. I found a confidence and worth that didn't depend on how others treated me. Now, when someone lashes out or lets me down, I can see that it's about them, not me. And when I feel triggered, I know it's an opportunity to heal something within myself.

I used to hate that saying, "It is better to have loved and lost than never to have loved at all." My heartbreak always wanted to argue against it. But now, I think I get it. It's about learning to hold both the beauty and the pain at the same time. Too often, our fear of being hurt keeps us from embracing the beautiful. Yet, in the end, that fear itself is the true thief—the one that brings the greatest loss.

We are meant to be in relationship with one another. Our brains are literally wired for community and belonging—that part isn't optional. What *is* optional is how we choose to show up. We can let past wounds keep us small and guarded, or we can take the risk of opening ourselves to love again.

And that's the thing about risk. If we never step toward the tree, we might avoid getting pooped on, but we'd also miss out on the special moments of connecting with the birds up close, seeing them from a unique perspective. We'd miss the chance to marvel at their small, fleeting beauty.

Yes, I got pooped on today. But I also got to watch the miracle of a little flock of birds take flight, and for a moment, it was breathtaking.

I chuckled for a few minutes as I cleaned up, (I should have taken a picture, but I'm sure you can imagine it!) and then I set out to enjoy the adventure of the rest of my day.

I hope wherever you are today, you're finding your own moments of messy beauty. And if a bird ever poops on your head, I hope you laugh as hard as I did.

All poop aside, know I'm sending my love,

- *L*

27. *Just Have Fun*

I have to tell you about something incredible I saw today. On my walk, just as I was heading back toward the house, a bird in the sky caught my attention. At first, I thought it was a hawk—majestic, soaring effortlessly, as they do. But then I noticed its solid black feathers. It was a raven.

What held my gaze, though, wasn't just the bird itself—it was the circus-style aerobatics it performed in the air. I have never seen anything like this before. I've seen hawks tuck and dive when going after their prey, but this was different. The raven would soar, then suddenly fold its wings and roll into a dive, twisting through the air before catching the wind again and lifting into another effortless glide. Over and over, it repeated this daring acrobatic dance.

At one point, something dropped from its beak—a leaf. I watched as it tucked its wings, plummeted toward the ground, and then, just before reaching it, snatched the leaf back up, and rose to soar again. I had never seen anything like it. This bird was *playing*. It wasn't hunting or trying to survive—it was simply enjoying the experience of flight and play.

Later, I learned that ravens are known for their playful nature. They'll carry objects high in the air, drop them, and dive after them just for fun. No agenda. No purpose. Just joy in the moment.

And it made me wonder: when did we forget how to play?

Lately, I've been reading a lot about loss, grief, and change. Heavy and necessary topics, but not much about the value of just *having fun*. So, I decided to start paying attention to the play around me. I watched the dogs at the park, leaping and tumbling without any apparent self-consciousness. I saw children making silly faces, running in circles, laughing for no reason. They weren't worried about productivity or whether their joy was justified. They just played.

Somewhere along the way, we stopped doing that. We got older, took on responsibilities, and convinced ourselves that play was a luxury we could no longer afford. We drowned in to-do lists, in expectations, in the weight of being an "adult." I once read that a four-year-old laughs three hundred times a day, while a forty-year-old only laughs four. I don't know if these numbers are exactly accurate, but the reality they reflect is hard to ignore.

And for people like you and me who have battled addiction, playfulness is often the first thing to disappear. At first, alcohol seemed like a shortcut to fun, a way to loosen up, to feel free. But that was a lie. A cruel one. Instead of bringing joy, it slowly siphoned it away.

What most people don't realize is that alcohol actually reduces the brain's ability to produce dopamine and serotonin—those very chemicals responsible for feeling happy, motivated, and at peace. The more we drink, the less of these chemicals our brains make on their own. That's why, over time, drinking stops being fun. The highs become duller, and the lows become deeper. Anxiety creeps in where joy used to be. Depression tightens its grip. The very thing we once relied on to feel good becomes the reason we feel worse. We've talked before about how alcohol also shrinks the prefrontal cortex—the part of the brain responsible for problem-solving, spontaneity, and *playfulness*. It literally stifles creativity, numbs curiosity, and kills the ability to experience real, unfiltered joy. No wonder everything felt heavy. No wonder laughter faded.

Of course, it's not only people with substance addictions who suffer from the lack of play and joy in everyday life. It seems like we as a society have put so much pressure on ourselves and others to always be respectful, responsible, and productive. Life becomes so much about duty and obligation that playfulness gets snuffed out. You and I often discussed how sad it was that when we would ask our clients what they do for fun, 99% of them responded with little to nothing.

But here's the beautiful part: just as our brains can be damaged, they can also heal. Laughter, play, and creativity aren't just luxuries—they're essential. Neuroscience tells us that play boosts dopamine, relieves stress, strengthens social bonds, and even helps the brain form new healthy pathways. Laughter lowers cortisol, improves circulation, and literally strengthens the immune system. The oxytocin it releases supports energy regulation for better sleep and emotional balance. Joy isn't frivolous—it's medicine.

I see this when I'm with my kids and grandkids. With them, play is effortless. We dance around the living room, singing ridiculous songs at the top of our lungs. We splash in the pool, chase each other through the park, play games, and laugh until our stomachs hurt—all for the sole purpose of having fun and connecting over the joy of play. They remind me of what the raven already knows.

If you were here right now, I would challenge you to a game of cribbage. Who knows, maybe I would even let you win…but not likely! Either way, I know we'd laugh our way through it.

For now, play well, my friend—and know I'm sending my love,

- L

28. What a Mess

I can see you now—shaking your head, smirking, maybe even laughing—
if you were here to witness the state of my bedroom and the rest of the
house. Clothes, books, musical instruments scattered everywhere! My
creativity may be one of my greatest strengths, but it comes with a
downside: I can be incredibly messy and disorganized. Things are almost
always out of order. And while I can ignore the chaos for a while,
eventually, it catches up with me. The clutter builds, the overwhelm sets in,
and suddenly, the thought of cleaning feels like an impossible mountain to
climb.

This is in direct contrast to someone like you, who instinctively tidies as
you go—putting things away after you get them out, wiping things down
immediately, keeping everything in order, and preventing messes from
accumulating in the first place. It always amazed me how effortless that
seemed for you—so natural. For me, it has always been a struggle.

It wasn't until recently that I was formally diagnosed with ADHD. Not that
it was a surprise to anyone who knows me well—including you. My
version of ADHD isn't the external hyperactivity that people typically
imagine. My hyperactivity is all internal: racing thoughts, restless energy,
emotional chaos. And you know what's fascinating? Research shows a
strong link between ADHD and addiction. Dr. Gabor Maté, one of the
leading experts in addiction, even titled a chapter in his book, *In the Realm
of Hungry Ghosts*, "Their Brains Never Had a Chance." He describes how
ADHD is a major risk factor for addiction—not just to substances like
nicotine, alcohol, and cocaine, but also to gambling, compulsive behaviors,
and other forms of self-medicating.

That certainly resonates with me. The constant sense of overwhelm I felt in
my life was one of the biggest triggers for my drinking. At first, I didn't
recognize the connection—after all, I had managed my anxiety and stress
without alcohol for years. But once I started drinking, my brain learned
quickly that alcohol offered a shortcut to relief. Of course, that shortcut
was actually a trap, but I didn't realize I was getting taken until I was
already deep in it.

ADHD affects the brain's dopamine system—our natural "reward" center. People with ADHD have lower baseline dopamine levels, which makes it harder for us to feel a sense of satisfaction, motivation, or "okay-ness." This is why we often seek stimulation or novelty—our brains are constantly craving that missing chemical boost. And guess what artificially floods the brain with dopamine? Alcohol. Drugs. Risk-taking. But here's the kicker: over time, substances don't just *supplement* our deficient dopamine levels—they *deplete* the baseline even further. They hijack the system, tricking the brain into relying on the substance rather than producing dopamine naturally.

And it isn't just dopamine. Chronic alcohol use also disrupts serotonin levels—the chemical that stabilizes mood. So, while I drank to escape anxiety or stress, in the long run, my drinking was making my anxiety and depression *worse*. The very thing I thought was helping me cope was actually robbing me of the ability to cope at all.

I wish you were here to talk about all of this in person—I can almost hear you teasing me, calling it another excuse. But you have to admit, it's a damn good one. And I know you get it. Maybe not the ADHD part, but everything else.

Of course, ADHD isn't *all* bad. In fact, I believe it is more than just a disorder—it's a different way of being in the world. When I worked with kids who had ADHD, I always reminded them that they had superpowers: heightened creativity, sharp intuition, deep sensitivity, and an incredible ability to notice details others overlook. Many of us are natural problem-solvers, quick thinkers, and great at connecting with people. But the challenge is that we live in a society built for neurotypical brains—ones that thrive on structure, predictability, and linear thinking. For someone like me, that structure can feel suffocating. And yet, without some level of order, life can quickly spiral into chaos.

When I was in rehab, one of the daily expectations was to make our beds and have everything picked up by 9:00 a.m. At first, I rolled my eyes at the idea. But they explained that these small habits help restore a sense of control—something that addiction strips away. And they were right. At that point, my life felt completely out of control. I couldn't control my drinking. I couldn't control my emotions. I couldn't even control my own thoughts. But I *could* make my bed. I *could* take one small step toward reclaiming order.

Developing healthy routines has been one of the most powerful tools in my recovery. And while my house might still get messy, my *life* doesn't feel like a mess anymore. I will always be the playful, creative, slightly chaotic soul you know and love—but that doesn't mean I have to live in a constant state of disorder.

Did I ever show you the prescription Dr. Bob, one of AA's founders, would give his patients? They gave it to us in rehab:

1. Trust God.
2. Clean house.
3. Help others.

Simple, but profound.

Trust God. To me, this means trusting not just in a higher power, but in the people and tools that have been put in place to help—treatment centers, medications, support groups, loving friends. It's about recognizing that I don't have to do this alone.

Clean house. This isn't just about physical clutter (though, I'm learning that a clean space does wonders for my mental state). It's also about letting go of anything that no longer serves me: the negative thought patterns, the old identities, the shame and self-judgment that kept me trapped in cycles of self-destruction. Cleaning out the internal garbage makes room for healing.

Help others. This one surprised me the most. I always thought I had to be "fixed" before I could offer anything to others—especially in the realm of addiction. But the truth is, helping others is *part* of that healing. Even small acts of kindness—offering a listening ear, showing up for a friend, and volunteering—pull us out of self-focus and connect us to something bigger. And connection is what ultimately saves us.

Speaking of *cleaning house,* I just took a break from writing to actually clean my house. (Shocking, I know.) And you know what? It feels amazing. It's funny how external order can bring such internal peace. Now, I think I'll celebrate my clean space with a cup of coffee and a slice of pie.

Wish you were here to join me!

As always, sending my love,

- *L*

29. The Child Within

This morning, I had a beautiful group session with one of my favorite mentors. We were talking about the purpose of life, and he shared a profound truth: *our purpose is to nurture the inner child within us.* To love that child unconditionally and allow it to grow in a safe, supportive space. We discussed how essential it is to bring our inner child into every experience—to let it see, learn, and adapt. To hold it close through life's ups and downs, offering the tenderness and safety it always deserved.

His words reminded me of a beautiful line from *The Shack,* a movie we watched the other night. There's a moment where Papa (God) points to a bird soaring in the sky and tells Mack, "That bird's purpose is to fly. Your purpose is to be loved." That really resonated with me—like a song coursing through my veins.

I believe that includes loving ourselves—not just receiving love from others or seeking it from God or the universe, but truly allowing ourselves to be loved and believing we are worthy of it. Yet, for so long, I didn't.

The thing is, while I was stuck in my addictive behaviors and thinking, it seemed I was much better at either pitying or despising my inner child. Even before drinking, shame distorted my reasoning, and I resented my inner child, often blaming it for my childhood wounds. My rational mind knew the child was innocent, but shame polluted the rational mind and overshadowed reason.

If we despise that innermost part of us, it is like having a cracked and unstable foundation. Everything else we try to build or become throughout our lives will, in some way, be unstable. If we are unable to love and believe in the innocence of our core being, we will struggle to adequately love or receive love from others.

This shame and convoluted thinking became increasingly more difficult as I became an adult. While I still made some good choices, the bad ones finally landed me in the depths of alcoholism, which nullified (in my mind) any of the good. It was hard, if not impossible, to imagine a sweet, innocent, loving child—much less embrace her.

Therapists often talk about the voices in our heads—the ones that don't belong to us, but rather to our parents, teachers, employers, or peers. You and I have compared notes about the ones that continue to whisper criticism, judgment, or blame, even long after those who first spoke them are gone. We adopt their voices as our own, holding ourselves to impossible standards, demanding perfection, and shaming ourselves when we fall short. Before long, there is little thought of embracing the inner heart of the child—gently and with kindness.

What makes things more challenging is when religion preaches that we are born sinners—evil and unworthy of even God's love. This kind of doctrine made it even harder for me to believe my inner child was worthy of the love she desperately needed. As I have grown in my own spiritual wisdom, as well as in the studies of biblical scripture and other resources, I know everyone is deeply loved, worthy, innocent, and embraced by the Author of Love. Even me.

If we could see ourselves the way a beloved child deserves to be seen— with patience, tenderness, and encouragement—how different would life feel? Instead of looking in the mirror with criticism, we would look with compassion. Instead of punishing ourselves for mistakes, we would guide ourselves with love. Instead of expecting perfection, we would allow ourselves to be human—learning, growing, and trying again.

I agree with my mentor that loving this innocent and divine inner child is the first step toward becoming my highest and most authentic self. And the more I reflect, the more I realize that, in the vast timeline of existence—the age of the earth, the wisdom of the universe—humanity is still young. We are children, still learning, still trying to figure it all out. If we consider the concept of an ever-evolving universe, then compared to God, the earth, and even the plants and animals that have roamed this world for far longer than we have, we humans are the newcomers. Perhaps if we embraced that truth, we could allow ourselves more grace, replacing rigid expectations with a childlike sense of wonder and curiosity. Maybe then, we would notice more of life's everyday miracles—the astonishing truths and quiet beauty we've long stopped seeing.

Can you see your own inner child? Mine is bright-eyed and full of wonder, playful and imaginative. She is sensitive, but strong. She is full of

106

curiosity, eager to learn, hopeful, and trusting. She is sacred. She deserves to be held, loved, and encouraged through all that lies ahead. And I intend to do just that.

For the record, I have always seen the beautiful, precious child within you. So, from my inner child to yours...

- *L*

30. *Spiritual Being*

Today, as I was rearranging some books on the shelf in my art room, a paper from my rehab binder fell out, landing by my feet. Isn't it funny how little signs like this show up exactly when we need them?

I know I've told you before how much I hated introducing myself at AA meetings by saying, "Hi, I'm L, and I am an alcoholic." It never sat right with me. Inside, I knew that wasn't my *identity*. It wasn't *who* I was—it was something I struggled with, something I was healing from, but not something that defined my soul.

That's why, when this paper landed in front of me today, I breathed out a sigh of gratitude. It was from a session our spiritual counselor led in rehab, the one where he shared his own journey with addiction and faith. Integrating Native American and Catholic influences, he offered a perspective that completely changed how I saw myself.

He said, "I am a spiritual being having a human experience, and my human body struggles with addiction to drugs and alcohol."

That hit home. Finally, an introduction that felt right. A way to acknowledge my struggle without letting it define me. It wasn't about being in denial. It was about separating the "who" from the "what."

For some people, even the word *spiritual* feels uncomfortable, like it comes with a contract to subscribe to a specific religious doctrine. I get it. I've talked with so many people who avoided AA because of the whole *Higher Power* thing, or who cringed when someone tried to talk to them about God. I've also met plenty who had faith at one point, but walked away after being wounded by religious institutions.

But here's the thing—most of us struggling with addiction don't get out of it alone. Addiction is bigger than we are. It is relentless. It will disguise itself as comfort, as relief, as an old friend who just wants to take the edge off. But in reality, it is the big bad wolf, ready to devour.

I do believe that overcoming such a consuming nemesis requires something greater than ourselves. However, I don't think that "something" has to fit into a neat little box labeled with one particular religion or belief system. Whether we call it God, Source, Creator, Spirit, Love—whatever resonates—it doesn't matter. What matters is that we find a power that grounds us, strengthens us, and pulls us out of the darkness.

I had my own spiritual foundation before addiction took hold, but I still had crisis moments. I was angry at God. Angry at how much I had suffered. Angry that I had to fight this addiction when I had spent my whole life trying to be a good person. Angry that, despite everything I'd tried to do right, my life kept crumbling. I felt abandoned.

But looking back, I see the truth. God didn't abandon me—I abandoned myself.

My shame and self-disgust-built walls so high, I refused to let God in. I sentenced myself to suffering, convinced I wasn't worthy of grace.

Yet somehow, despite it all, I was still delivered. And not in some dramatic, miraculous moment—but through the grit of recovery. Through a rehab program that forced me to do the hard work. Through the people who supported me. Through the slow and steady process of rebuilding my life. Through remembering that I was more than just my addiction and continually reconnecting to my spiritual self. That was the real miracle.

I wish more people understood that spirituality isn't about religion. Religion *can* be a beautiful way to practice spirituality, or it can be a rigid box that suffocates it. For me, faith has never been about checking the right doctrinal boxes. It has been about love—a pure, unconditional, *no matter what you've done or where you've been* kind of love.

You and I have talked so many times about how people get caught up in defining God, like God could fit into a neat little theological box. But if we're talking about an infinite being, doesn't it make sense that our finite minds might struggle to grasp it all? That's why we have so many religions, so many different ways of seeking and understanding the Divine. But at the core, the message is the same: *Love. Connection. Healing.*

My dad often comes to mind when I wrestle with these thoughts. You know how stubborn he was. He had all the classic arguments against faith—the hypocrisy, the suffering, the illogic of it all. But I'll never forget when he admitted to me, with tears in his eyes, that he *couldn't not believe* in God. Even with all his objections, something inside him just knew.

And that's the thing. I believe we *all* know. We can argue and resist, we can call it by different names, but there's something within us that longs for that connection, that love that's bigger than anything we can manufacture ourselves.

One of my favorite questions to ask clients who are struggling to believe in their worthiness is: *"In the very beginning, what material did the Creator have to work with?"* The answer? *Only the Divine Creator.* Which means everything—every tree, every ocean, every star, every person—is made of divine material. *We* are made of divine material.

The same minerals found in human DNA are found in the stars. The same molecular structures exist in plants, animals, and the human body. This is either an amazing coincidence or we are literally what I call "God-stuff."

So, what does that make us? Divine. Sacred. Worthy.

And if we are made of divine material, how could we ever be unworthy? How could we ever be too far gone? So, I'll leave you with this, my friend—something I say now with confidence, peace, and clarity:

> I am a spiritual being, having a human experience.

> My human body is in recovery from addiction to alcohol.

And that's not something to be ashamed of. It's something to be proud of. Goodnight, my fellow God-stuff friend.

As always, sending my love.

- *L*

31. *Drunk Dream*

Last night, I had another drunk dream. It is so discombobulating. It's been a while, but it still rattles me every time it happens. I wake up feeling unsettled, guilty—almost hungover—until I fully come to my senses and realize, with immense relief, *it was just a dream.* Even knowing how common these are in recovery, the disorienting effects linger, like a shadow of the past trying to creep back in.

In the dream, I was at a party—one of *those* parties. The kind where people drink, let loose, and cross the line from fun into reckless. I felt the familiar tingles of excitement, that rush of anticipation, my pulse quickening at the thought of a drink in my hand. The strangest part? In this dream, I believed that *this time* I could drink like other people. That somehow, the rules had changed, and I could enjoy alcohol without consequence.

And then, there was him. A young man I once knew—one who went into rehab a month after me. Always the life of the party, larger than life itself. If anyone was going to justify my drinking, it was him. But instead, he looked me in the eyes and gently, but firmly, said, "L, today is a really important day for you to stay sober. Today is not a good day to drink."

I remember the disappointment that swept over me in the dream. But when I woke up, his words resonated in a way I didn't expect. *Today is a good day to be sober. Today is always a good day to be sober.*

These dreams remind me of a truth I sometimes wish I could forget: there is a part of me that will always be powerless against alcohol. That part doesn't just disappear because I've abstained for years. On bad days, when stress, grief, or exhaustion creep in, my first thought is still, *I want a drink.* Not *I should call a friend,* or *I need to go for a walk,* or *I should pray.* Those come second, third—maybe fourth. But the first impulse is always the same. And that is the nature of addiction.

While I am in my recovery, I know that, on one level, I have gained victory over my alcoholism. This victory is powerful, but it is conditional. Success over the addiction is only success as long as I don't take a drink.

It's also the essence of Step One: admitting we are powerless over alcohol and that our lives have become unmanageable. I've struggled with that step—*powerlessness* feels too much like *helplessness*. And I don't do well with helplessness.

We both know what it's like to be young children in situations that should never happen to a child. That kind of helplessness is real. And when those experiences happen repeatedly throughout childhood, it becomes something deep and enduring—a learned helplessness. It stops being an event and becomes a way of being. A pattern of expecting that no matter what we do, things won't change—so why try?

It's not just psychological, either. Physiologically, early trauma actually changes the way our brains develop. You may or may not know this yet, but the medial prefrontal cortex—the part of the brain tied to our identity, decision-making, and a sense of self—becomes compromised. This literally increases our vulnerability or "predisposition" for addiction. It's not about personal weakness. It's about biology.

Add to this the reality that each of us also tends to look for evidence that will confirm our worst fears or pre-existing beliefs—whatever they are. If we believe or fear that we are helpless, we will subconsciously find circumstances or situations in which we *are* helpless or feel helpless, reinforcing that belief. It's a kind of cruel self-validation, convincing us that we truly have no agency, even in situations where we do.

True, sometimes helplessness *is* real. There are moments when we simply *cannot* change a situation. When a loved one is dying, when a pet is suffering, when a natural disaster strikes—we cannot bargain, fight, or outsmart these things. And yet, we still find ourselves trying. We tell ourselves we *should* be able to do something, to fix it, to stop the suffering, to prevent the loss. And when we can't, we feel like failures.

Many of us carry this subconscious expectation that we should be able to in some way change *everything*—that if we just try harder, love more, push past the pain, we can bend reality to our will. But some things are simply unchangeable. And that truth can be deeply unsettling.

To navigate the tension between powerlessness and helplessness, I have been working to embrace the power and simplicity of the Serenity Prayer, which I know you have heard me rattle off numerous times. Still, it's worth repeating:

> God, grant me the serenity to accept the things I cannot change,
> The courage to change the things I can,
> And the wisdom to know the difference.

It's simple, but it's not easy. Accepting that some things—pain, loss, other people's actions—are outside my control goes against everything in me. The desire to change, to fix, to prevent suffering is so strong. At the same time, I am also learning that finding *courage* to act where I am *not* helpless is just as important as the serenity of acceptance.

While I can't control everything, I *can* take action where it matters. If I have the ability to make a difference, I *can choose* to do something. If I see someone being harmed, I *can choose* to intervene. Free will allows people to make terrible choices, but it also gives *me* the choice to stand up, to step in, to make a change where I can.

And where I can't—when I'm just an observer of something I wish I could fix—I've decided to act in another way: through prayer, through intention, through sending love and healing energy into the world. Maybe that sounds small, but I don't think it is. I truly believe in the power of prayer, of sending blessings, of holding space for others in their suffering. Maybe I can't always act externally, but I can always take action *internally.*

In that respect, there can actually be action within the inaction. There is a true power within. You and I, along with everyone else, can tap into it when we feel powerless on the outside. This is how I find my grounding and strength when things like drunk dreams or negative news begin to plague my mind.

So, maybe I *am* powerless over alcohol. But I am *not* powerless in life. I am not helpless. I have choices, strength, and wisdom.

And today—just like yesterday, just like tomorrow—*is* a good day to be sober.

Sending my love...

- *L*

32. *Thank you!*

Thank you! Thank you! Thank you!

I owe you more "thank yous" than I can count. Over the years, there have been so many moments, so many things you did, said, or gave that I never adequately thanked you for. And now, I realize how few true thank-you notes I've actually written in my whole life—beyond the occasional text or a rushed "Thanks" in passing. It's an important practice, and one I intend to do more of moving forward. There's something powerful about pausing to acknowledge gratitude in a tangible way. Taking the time to sit down, write a note, or even make a call requires being fully present in the act of appreciation.

I like to think I'm good at pausing to appreciate the beauty in nature—a stunning sunset, a rainbow after a storm, or the rare moment when a wild animal crosses my path. Those moments feel sacred, and I let myself soak them in. But when it comes to the people in my life, too often I recognize the blessing and then rush right past it—like a car speeding through a breathtaking landscape without stopping to take it in. I notice, I feel grateful, and then, just as quickly, I move on.

I can practically hear you smirking now, squinting your eyes and saying, *"I've never received a thank-you note from you."* And you'd be right. But hey, like I said, it's a new intention, and I'm working on it. Here's what I'm learning: when I take the time to truly express gratitude—to write the note, return the kind act, or speak the words out loud—it doesn't just bless the person receiving it. This loving interaction blesses *me* as well.

As you know, it's so easy for me to get caught up in the noise—the distractions, the worries, the endless list of things that could go wrong. Inflation, politics, natural disasters, relationship struggles, grief...oh, and let's not forget the basement flooding. (Yes, that just happened.) The negative things in life are loud. They demand attention. They barge in uninvited and make themselves at home.

But when I choose to shift my focus—when I intentionally look for something to be grateful for—it changes everything. Gratitude doesn't erase the hard things, but it offers a counterbalance. It reminds me that beauty still exists, even in the midst of challenges.

For me, gratitude has been a *lifeline* in sobriety. Most of the drinks I ever took were paired with some kind of excuse that focused on the negative. A bad day at work, an argument, financial stress, the weather—whatever it was, I could always find a reason to drown my sorrows. Alcohol was my way of numbing, of avoiding, of escaping. But at its core, it was also a reflection of what I was focusing on.

I've come to understand that what I *choose* to focus on impacts the way I experience life. The brain, after all, functions in networks. When I'm having a bad day and focusing on what's wrong, what I call my "negative network" gets activated, lighting up all the associated emotions, memories, and perspectives. Suddenly, *everything* feels worse. But practicing gratitude—even for the smallest things—helps strengthen my "positive network." And with time, it has actually made *joy* easier for me to access.

Now that my mind and body are healthier, I get to choose how I show up in each moment. I can choose what I focus on. And today, I choose gratitude. So, in this moment—this one right here, which I hear you whispering *"is the only moment"*—I want to say…

Thank you.
Thank you for every way you've been there for me, for everything you've given, for the ways you still help me from afar. Thank you for the laughter, the lessons, the love, and even the hard moments that helped me grow. Thank you for being *you*.
~As always, sending my love.

- *L*

33. *Healer*

Last week, I had a new and unexpected experience. At a conference exhibit, I wandered over to a stand where an Indian woman was offering Henna—those beautiful, temporary, hand-painted tattoos. I figured, *why not?* As she carefully traced intricate designs onto my palms, she offered a blessing. Then she looked up at me and said, "You are a healer. It doesn't matter what you do; healing is simply who you are."

Her words settled deep within me. I wasn't surprised, not at this point in my life, but still, it felt affirming. Sometimes, I get so caught up in the *how*—what modality, what technique, what method—I forget that healing isn't about *how* as much as it's about *why*. The *why* has always been clear: to help people find hope, moving toward health and wholeness.

I've been thinking a lot about healing lately, especially seeing so much suffering in this overstimulated, high-pressure, conflict-ridden world. So many people are barely hanging on, trying to manage their pain or numb themselves with junk food, pills, alcohol, or a thousand other distractions—knowing, deep down, these things only mask the real issues. They might offer a moment of relief, but ultimately, they create a deeper wound.

Healing, though, isn't just one prescribed path. It's not a single medicine, a single therapy, a single belief system. Healing is a vast, open field. It's fluid, much like water—ever-changing, ever-flowing, taking the form it needs depending on the circumstance. As I walked beside the river today, I found myself reflecting on all the ways water reflects the nature of healing.

Rain soothes us to sleep. Snow blankets the earth, offering quiet permission to rest. The ocean reminds us of vastness and mystery—hidden treasures beyond what we can see. Rivers carve new paths over time, purifying and reshaping the land, just as healing reshapes us. Even fog, with its quiet stillness, reminds us that we are sometimes suspended between worlds—between seasons, between transformations, between knowing and not knowing. And then there's the rainbow—a symbol of hope, a whisper that even after the storm, there is beauty.

Healing comes in many forms, and I know we've both practiced countless modalities. The way I see it, each modality offers unique benefits. Traditional talk therapy addresses the cognitive, conscious mind, helping people process their present experiences. EMDR and clinical hypnosis allow for deeper subconscious healing. Breathwork therapies activate the body's natural healing processes and release stored tension. And medical psychotropics, when used appropriately, can alter states of consciousness to aid recovery of deep-seated trauma.

Then there are creative expressions—art therapy, play therapy, music therapy—offering insight and transformation in ways that words alone cannot. Energy practices like Reiki, Qigong, chakra balancing, and vibrational healing through sound (something I now practice with my Tibetan bowls) can facilitate profound physical and emotional effects. I've even been exploring and learning about the properties of gemstones and how they might be used therapeutically.

Then, of course, there are the healers who work directly with the body— doctors, nurses, physical therapists, chiropractors, acupuncturists, and massage therapists—each playing a vital role in restoring movement, function, and health. And let's not forget the indigenous medicine people— the shamans and traditional healers—who see illness as not merely a physical condition, but rather a deeper imbalance within the spiritual, emotional, and energetic realms. Through sacred ceremonies and ancestral healing traditions, they seek to restore harmony and well-being on every level.

It's a gift to live in a time where we have access to such an abundance of healing methods. At the same time, I always remind my clients that finding the right approach is like finding the right pair of shoes—it has to fit. It has to support you, feel comfortable, and align with where you are in your journey.

Of course, even the most skilled healers cannot help someone who isn't *willing* to receive healing. That was a hard lesson for me to learn. I remember the shame and suffocating sense of failure when I finally had to admit that I couldn't overcome my addiction on my own. As a therapist—a *healer*—I should have been able to heal myself, right? At least, that's what my shame kept telling me. The "shoulds" were relentless.

The shame and humiliation were exactly what I was drowning in at that point. Still, it was absolutely necessary for me to get to this place of being willing to *receive*—to let someone else hold space for me, guide me, and help me find my way back to myself. All the healing tools in the world would have been useless if I had remained closed off, unwilling to let them in.

Then I learned about the *nocebo effect*. We all know about the placebo effect—how the belief in healing amplifies its effectiveness. But fewer people talk about its opposite: nocebo, where the belief that something *won't* work actually blocks healing from occurring. It's not just psychological; there are real physiological effects.

There are documented cases where individuals were misdiagnosed with a terminal illness, only to develop symptoms or some other illness and die within the expected timeline—despite never having had the disease to begin with. That's how powerful belief is. The mind-body connection is undeniable.

The experience of needing help—*really* needing it—humbled me in ways I couldn't have anticipated. It shattered the illusion that I was somehow separate from the very design of life itself. Nature flourishes through interconnection. No creature exists in isolation. Healing, like life, is a *shared* experience.

Releasing the illusion of self-sufficiency, breaking free from the ego's need to be the healer rather than the one undergoing healing, has given me more peace than I ever thought possible. Now, whether I am offering healing or receiving it, I do so with open hands.

Tonight, I am offering a sound healing session with my new Tibetan bowls. The vibrations will fill the space, shifting the energy, carrying intention and resonance. I wish you could be here, sitting across from me, feeling the waves of sound ripple through your being. Instead, I'll simply send them to you across time and space.

As always, sending my love.

- *L*

34. The Sound of Silence

I chuckle as I think of all the conferences and trainings we went to together where we were told—sometimes repeatedly—to quiet down. We have always been quite the talkers when we've gotten together! And of course, I can still hear the voices from my childhood, telling me to "sit down and stop talking."

Silence is one of those things I both love and hate.

Today, when I'm out in nature, silence feels sacred—it allows me to hear everything else more clearly: the wind rustling through trees, the rhythmic splash of a river, the hum of unseen insects. But when silence has been forced upon me—when someone has refused to speak to me or when I've been shut out from connection—it has felt oppressive, suffocating, unbearable.

For years, I was so uncomfortable with silence, not because I didn't appreciate it, but because I wasn't comfortable being fully present in my own body, my own thoughts, and my own emotions. Silence left me alone with myself, and I wasn't sure I wanted that company.

I remember struggling with long pauses in conversation, feeling the overwhelming urge to fill the space, to "move things along." But now I understand: those quiet moments aren't empty—they're full. That's when the whispers of intuition and wisdom have a chance to be heard. You and I have talked about this often, The "power of the pause," as we like to call it—how intentional silence can be a source of insight rather than discomfort.

Recently, I had two very different experiences that illustrated this contrast between liberating silence and oppressive silence.

The first was in Sedona, Arizona, when I treated myself to a personal retreat. There, silence felt expansive. It wasn't just the absence of noise; it was the presence of stillness. I hiked alone, greeted strangers on the trail when I wanted to, and occasionally filled the air with my own sound—

playing my singing bowls or humming softly to myself, all while feeling deeply connected to the earth beneath me.

Then there was the monastery in New Mexico. When I arrived, I imagined I would have a similarly peaceful experience—one where I could practice silence when I felt drawn to it. Instead, I was met with a rigidly enforced rule: no talking with other guests. Meals were silent, and instead of fostering mindfulness, this forced hush only created discomfort. People avoided eye contact, staring at their plates as if even looking at one another was a violation.

Can you imagine my inner rebellious teenager's reaction? I hear you laughing now!

Of course, while we were silenced, the natural world refused to obey. The bees hummed wildly in the fields, birds sang, owls called to one another across the canyon at night. It was as if nature itself was reminding me: silence is not meant to stifle—it is meant to expand.

These contrasting experiences made me think about the different types of space we allow ourselves. The fishbowl versus the open pond. The potted plant versus the wild-growing tree.

We grow in accordance with the space we're given—or the space we claim.

For so many years, I felt trapped. I believed I was confined by my circumstances, by obligations, by expectations I didn't think I could challenge. That feeling of being stuck created frustration, resentment, and eventually, numbing. Drinking became my escape from the circumstances—the silence—I didn't know how to sit with.

The irony, of course, was that alcohol was its own form of silence. It shut down my emotions instead of helping me process them. It dulled my senses, disconnected me from my body, and left me imprisoned in a mental fog. I would justify to myself that I was drinking to "break free" or escape, but really, I was drinking to stay small.

And here's what I now understand: nothing was actually trapping me. I wasn't confined by my marriage, my career, my responsibilities, or the expectations of others. The real oppressor was the *belief* that I was trapped. The false idea that I had no choice.

Through all my healing, I have realized I am not a victim of my circumstances—I am the one who shapes them. I choose how I engage with my world. I choose whether I stay quiet or speak up. I choose whether I feel caged or free. The monastery felt oppressive because I let it feel that way—just as I created the beautiful experience of silence in Sedona.

I remember when we read *Man's Search for Meaning* together. Victor Frankl, a Holocaust survivor, wrote:

> Everything can be taken from a man but one thing: the last of the human freedoms—to choose one's attitude in any given set of circumstances, to choose one's own way…Between stimulus and response there is a space. In that space is our power to choose our response. In our response lies our growth and freedom.

This is a liberating truth worth remembering. Believing this, I have been able to place myself into bigger and better situations and environments that allow growth. I can find rest in silence, and I can choose to break it when I need to. I no longer wish to live a life I feel the need to escape from. There are always choices and options. I truly am free to create whatever life I want to have.

So, here's to the beautiful, spacious sound of silence!

As always, sending my love,

• *L*

35. Running Together

Today was a walk down memory lane—or rather a memory "track." Did you ever make it to one of my son's track meets? I remember sitting on the edge of my seat watching, cheering, and anticipating which budding athlete would cross the finish line first. Well, I walked a similar track today, and I noticed they actually have short lines painted in each lane to let the relay runner know when it is time to pass the baton. It struck me how much clearer the transition is when the markers are visible, when there's a guide that says, *Now. Now is the time to let go and trust the next runner to carry forward.*

It would be nice if life had such clear markers, wouldn't it? While the memories of my boy's races brought a smile to my face, walking that track also brought up a more sorrowful memory.

A few months ago, my mother was lying in bed, unconscious, her body letting go in slow increments. But even as she drifted between worlds, I could tell she was struggling. She wasn't ready. She loved life too much to leave it behind easily.

I took her hand, feeling the lump in my throat rise. I whispered through my tears, "It's okay, Mom. We'll be alright." I wanted her to know that she didn't have to hold on for us, that she had done enough, that she could let go when she was ready.

I told her, "You can pass the baton to me, and I will do my best to continue the good work you started."

That moment has stayed with me. It made me think about my own mortality, my own sense of unfinished work.

I don't fear dying. I believe that something good awaits on the other side. But I do fear fading. I fear growing old and no longer having something valuable to offer. I fear feeling like a burden, like dead weight. In a culture that prioritizes youth and productivity, aging can feel like a slow erasure. To be "done" or retired is to be dismissed. I'm learning this is a common fear for those in the later years of life.

On reflection, I didn't only drink to escape a troubled youth or to cope with trauma I hadn't processed. My heaviest drinking started when life was passing me by, and it felt like my relevance was passing with it.

The perfect storm hit: my kids left home, menopause arrived with its mood swings and identity shifts, my back pain intensified, and the losses started piling up—family, friends, my sense of purpose. Aging was in my face and the fear of losing value and importance felt like a tightening grip around my throat. Alcohol softened the edges of that fear. Until, of course, it made everything worse.

The lifeline of therapists, mentors, and friends like you became essential during that dark time. You helped lay the groundwork for me to eventually see that growing older doesn't mean fading away—it means stepping into wisdom.

I know you've heard me talk about Parker Palmer's book, *On the Brink of Everything*. Did you ever get a chance to read it? He challenges the idea that elders should simply "pass the baton" and step aside. Instead, he invites us to join with one another in the race. He invites us to bring the wisdom of multiple generations to the table—or as he describes it, to the "orchestra." As he explains, "The elders help the young adults learn to play their instruments, and the younger generation helps the elders hear the emerging music of the world more clearly."

Isn't that a powerful shift in thinking?

In so many ways, our culture seems to get aging wrong. In past generations and in many indigenous cultures, and even in other present-day countries, elders are honored. Their wisdom is revered while they are still living. A person who has lived more years is respected more highly, invited in for guidance and instruction, instead of pushed out.

Today, we equate knowledge with wisdom, but they are not the same. Knowledge is data, gathered in books and online. Wisdom is lived experience, earned through trials and failures, heartbreak and healing. And wisdom needs a voice.

I think of my own journey—years of education, training, therapy work, and advanced certifications. The colors on my professional palette are varied, but my intuition—the wisdom I've gathered through practice and presence—is what guides my brush.

I could keep all of that to myself. Let it fade with me. Or I could share it. I could mentor young therapists. Walk alongside them instead of stepping aside. I could keep learning from them, too—because wisdom flows both ways. If I choose to be a part of an orchestra, joining with others from different generations who have the same passions, everyone's gifts are magnified and more complete.

Maybe the space between those white painted lines on the track needs to be longer. Or maybe that's me trying to hold on and not let the next generation run their own race. Maybe, instead of believing the world has left me behind, walking off the track, and turning to a bottle, I can find ways to still let those I've influenced move forward into their lives without disconnecting completely. Perhaps sometimes we're running our own races, sometimes we're cheering our loved-ones on from the stands, and sometimes we're playing our own parts alongside everyone else—bringing our own unique contributions and enriching one another, no matter our age. Things are constantly evolving—mindsets, culture, technology, expectations. There will never be a one-size-fits-all solution for life's challenges. But one thing remains the same: we need each other.

Wisdom deepens when it is shared. The younger professional generations may know the latest research, but the older generations know the deeper truths. And both are necessary. That realization shifts my perspective on aging. It allows me to move beyond the fear of fading and into the action of "saging." Though I told my mom it's okay to pass the baton, I still feel her wisdom with me, even now—as if she is writing this letter alongside me, whispering truths into my heart, reminding me that we are never really finished.
So, here's to aging well and sharing the baton—or music—so we can all add our own harmony to the melody of life!

Sending my love,

- *L*

36. Wings of Resilience

I wasn't expecting to see an eagle today. The snow from last night had covered everything in a crisp, silent white, and the open space felt entirely mine. My dog and I were enjoying our usual morning walk when I saw a large bird approaching. I assumed it was a hawk—after all, they're regulars around here. But as it got closer, I realized the unmistakable wingspan, the stark white head. A bald eagle! In ten years, I've never seen one in this area.

It soared directly over us and landed in a tree just ahead. My heart fluttered at the sight, and I stood there for a long moment, watching in awe. When we finally continued our walk, the eagle took off, circled around us as if marking our path, and returned to the same tree. I don't know why, but it felt like a special moment—one of those little nudges from the universe, reminding me to pay attention.

Noticing the dark clouds in the distance, I remembered there was a storm forecasted. This brought to mind an incredible story I heard about how the eagle deals with a storm. I was told that when a storm is approaching, the eagle flies directly into it, using the resistance of the powerful wind to propel itself to heights above the storm clouds. It was said that there were all types of ways the eagle's body adapted to allow it to stay above the storm until it passed. While it turns out that's a myth—eagles actually take cover like everyone else—the idea still resonates. How amazing would it be if we could rise above our problems like that, untouched by the chaos below?

Back when I was drinking, I didn't know how to filter all the chaos. Stress, conflict, fear—I absorbed it all until I was drowning in it. And I drank to quiet it. But now, I can see it for what it is—just noise. And I get to decide what deserves my attention.

Now, when I find myself having a particularly challenging day, I imagine sitting in the higher realms with my loving God. I work to stay above the day-to-day stressors of life—the societal pressures and fears that can really take over my thoughts and emotions, if I let them. Politics, family divisions, and work conflicts can create havoc within us. Media fuels fear to boost their ratings, even at the cost of spewing ugliness and hate. All of this creates a storm of uneasiness, despair, terror, and even war.

There is a scripture in the Bible that says we can "mount up with wings as eagles." I love the idea of using the wind of the storm to thrust me to higher places—soaring like the eagle above the negativity.

But let's be real. Some days, I don't feel like an eagle. Some days, I feel more like a duck, doing my best to keep from sinking. I expect you're smiling and nodding your head. But you know what? Ducks have their own kind of wisdom. They have a resiliency that is every bit as effective as the eagle metaphor.

When I was a school counselor, students would often come to me in tears, devastated by the hurtful words and actions of others. As I wiped their tears, I would gently encourage them to "make like a duck" and let it roll off their back. I would go on to explain how the duck uses its beak to stroke its feathers, which activates a special gland to release a special oily and waxy substance called sebum.

Oftentimes, when we observe them with their heads turned and twisted back, they are actually getting this oily substance onto their beak, then spreading it over their feathers and body. This "preening" waterproofs their exterior—an essential preparation for all the time they spend in the water. It also helps to rid the ducks of parasites and moisturizes their feathers so they can stay flexible, strong, and ready for flight. This is more *my* style— imagining myself as a duck while I engage in regular preening practices like prayer, music, walks in nature, setting necessary boundaries, and fostering intentional, positive communication with myself and those I love.

While there are countless opportunities for worry or frustration, it seems to me that much of the conflict and animosity between people is out of proportion. Honestly, the news is just too much for me these days. Truth be told, it is actually rare for me to read or watch it these days. I'd rather not fill my mind with stories of looting during natural disasters, rage-induced shootings on the highway, or the many other ways people hurt each other. I find I have to work to rise above thoughts that could consume me, and sometimes that means deciding not to seek them out. They too easily lead to a sort of mental chaos and self-destructive behavior, including drinking.

I recently heard this phrase, "Where attention goes, energy flows." So, I'm being careful where I put my focus!

There is also a proverb in the Bible that supports this idea: "Above all else, guard your heart, for everything you do flows from it." So instead of watching or reading things that will cause feelings of chaos and despair, I practice ways to "soar like an eagle" or "make like a duck." And in some ways, I think these two birds are practicing the same kind of skill.

Remember how we would talk about the imagination station, where we would use visualization meditations to relax? This is probably my best "preening tool." It can be so helpful to imagine myself soaring into a higher place of being or consciousness. There, I can feel more connected to the Creator, experiencing the presence of a higher love, and staying above all the disparaging things of this world that are out of my control.

Studies show that our bodies react to visualization techniques as though what we are imagining is real. Even the neural pathways respond as though we are having the actual physical experiences we imagine! We see this when we fear things or worry about things that haven't happened yet and probably will never happen. Still, the imagery we generate in fear can put our bodies into a state of distress as though what we feared is actually happening.

Fortunately, we can also create the opposite effect by imagining and visualizing beautiful, peaceful things like being in a safe, relaxing place or sitting in a temple with the Divine. When we imagine with the five senses—"noticing" what we see, hear, smell, taste and feel in that imaginary place—our bodies will physiologically respond as though we were actually there. Our blood pressure and heart rate lowers and our muscles relax. Levels of dopamine (the neurotransmitter of reward), serotonin (the neurotransmitter of happiness), and GABA (the neurotransmitter of calmness) all rise in response to meditations like these. In this dream-like state, we allow ourselves to experience a potential reality that becomes a sort of *actual* reality in our being.

Chaos has been in the world since the beginning of human existence, and it will continue long after I'm gone. I've learned that surviving—and potentially even thriving—in the midst of it is going to involve techniques such as these. By choosing to focus on higher things and understanding there is more at work here than what I can see or understand, I can face the storm and allow the strong winds blowing against me to thrust me to a higher place. I can trust there is a good outcome up ahead as I choose to believe the Author of Love is in charge. And when I don't feel like I can fly, I can still find peace. I can "preen" with loving self-care, knowing I don't have to fix it or understand it. In times like these, I can settle into a deep sense of calm, trusting that a higher power—my very life source—will carry out the work that needs to be done within and around me.

No more bad news for me today. Instead, I'm going to close my eyes and imagine you and me soaring together—or maybe just floating peacefully, feeling the warmth of the sun on our backs, hearing the distant lapping of water, the rustling of the trees... I like to think that's what real peace feels like—whether in the sky or on the water, carried by something bigger than us.

As always, sending my love...

- *L*

37. Hope vs. Expectations

You know me—the queen of expectations! My mother used to say, "Expectations are just premeditated resentments." She was right; expectations set me up for disappointment. Worse, they often lead to judgment. When someone doesn't meet my expectations, it's easy to focus on what they did wrong. And when I feel let down, I sometimes justify my disappointment by blaming them. Sadly, none of that has stopped me from having expectations.

During my drinking years, this cycle was my constant companion. My expectations for others were sky high, and when people inevitably let me down, frustration and aggravation bubbled over. It wasn't just disappointment—it was a bitter, gnawing anger. And you know what I did with that anger. I drank it down. Every unmet expectation became another excuse to pour a glass, which turned into a bottle, which turned into days I could barely remember.

The deeper I sank, the further hope slipped away from me. I stopped believing things could ever get better. Instead, I clung to control, grasping at it like a lifeline—if I could just *force* the world to meet my expectations, maybe I'd feel okay. But the harder I tried to control things, the more they spiraled, and the more I was drowning in my own despair.

Looking back, it's clear that losing hope was what really fueled my drinking. Without it, life felt like one big disappointment. I thought I could drink my way out of the pain, but instead, I drank my way deeper into it.

Hope and expectations are critically different, but I didn't understand that then. Both come from wanting something to turn out a certain way, but hope is trusting that things will work out, even if it's not how you planned. Expectations, on the other hand, are rigid. They demand control, and when control slips through your fingers (as it always does), expectations can leave you bitter, angry, and empty.

There's a Bible verse that says, "Now hope does not disappoint, because the love of God has been poured out in our hearts by the Holy Spirit who was given to us." While I could have quoted this to you word for word, for a long time, I didn't really believe it. I had built a wall so high with my expectations, frustrations, and shame that there was no room for hope to get in.

It wasn't until I began my journey to sobriety that I started to see the difference. I realized that my expectations of others were a reflection of the harsh expectations I had for myself. When I judged myself as unworthy, I judged others just as harshly. When they didn't meet my needs or my standards, I took it personally, as if their actions were proof of my own failure. But the more I recognize these tendencies in myself, the more I can work to change them. I now realize that judgment, high expectations, and the need for control all have the same root of shame. Deep down, I thought that if I couldn't control the world around me, it meant something was wrong with me.

Of course, life doesn't care about my need for control. The world refuses to revolve around my preferences, no matter how hard I try. (Rude, right?) So, I'm learning to let go. I'm trusting in a higher power—the source of love who sees what I can't—and working to stay in that divine flow.

While this comes with no expectation, know that I send this letter in authentic love with the hope that you are well, my dear friend.

- *L*

38. More Than the Sum

I was just thinking of all the times we used to discuss client cases, trying to make sense of their journeys. One of us would often say that we are all the "sum of our experiences." I suspect this idea was at the root of another wild dream I just had.

In the dream, I saw a person—representing me—standing beneath a huge, wide funnel hovering above my head. Inside the funnel were images of every experience I've ever had, swirling together—the traumas, the joys, the heartbreaks, the miracles. It was all there, from childhood wounds to moments of deep love, from failures to triumphs.

Then something strange happened. The funnel wasn't just collecting these experiences—it was refining them. Melting them down, breaking them apart, fusing them back together in a way that transformed them. The whole mass became a thick liquid—like molten metal—and slowly poured into my body.

I woke up thinking: this is what life does to us. We don't just carry our experiences, untouched, like rocks in a backpack. They shape us, integrate into us, refine us. I was reminded once again how important it is that we actually "process" and work through our experiences. Someone who just ignores the pains and hard times, or somehow escapes from emotions altogether, would have a different "sum" than one who leans in, walks through the fire, lets it burn away what it must, and emerges transformed.

Every situation is a valuable and important part of our life's journey and our soul's story. In rehab, we were taught about and walked the Medicine Wheel, a tool used by indigenous peoples for understanding the seasons and inevitable challenges that come and go throughout our lives.

This was a large circle, maybe twelve feet in diameter, that was formed using rocks the size of softballs. From the center of the circle, more stones extended to the perimeter in the shape of a cross, pointing North, East, South, and West. Learning about this tool gave me a framework for processing experiences I once thought abnormal or shameful with grace and strength.

The lessons of the Medicine Wheel are valuable because they explain how anything growing always grows as a system of circles and cycles. These "sacred circle" teachings are believed to align with a system that the Great Spirit put into place to share knowledge, information, and concepts. And within this framework, we are reminded that every moment is a sacred moment.

There are multiple ways in which the Medicine Wheel is used. In one method, each of the four directions represents different qualities, powers, challenges, and life experiences. Here, the wheel teaches about the cycle of life, starting in the east with new birth. Then, in the south, there is the direction of the youth. In the west is adulthood. And in the north, the elder.

There is also a wheel for seasons of the year, such as spring, summer, fall, and winter. Springtime is about new beginnings and possibilities. Summertime represents new, flourishing growth. Fall represents the time of bountiful harvest. Winter calls for a time to stop and reflect as Mother Earth rests. In this wheel, we see all the stages of life, like the cycle of the seasons, in a circular, ongoing pattern.

The Native Americans use the four directions to represent times of growth in the emotional, mental, physical, and spiritual realms. They believe that for true growth to be achieved, one must work within all four directions. In each of these directions, there are challenges and struggles, but they are balanced with positive experiences and strengths. It's a polarity-based system, divinely created to keep things in balance.

The Medicine Wheel doesn't teach denial or avoidance. It normalizes experiences and stresses the importance of movement through any situation. I see now how, for years, I fought against the wheel. Instead of flowing through the emotions, through the seasons, and through my pain, I drank to numb—and I got stuck.

Finally embracing what the Medicine Wheel had to offer has led me to another Native American teaching that, to be honest, I've struggled with. It states that we have the *choice* of living "in harmony" or "out of harmony," and that this choice determines the results in each stage of our development. For years, this was incredibly difficult to believe, because although I wanted harmony, my actions often created disharmony—both internally and externally. Clearly, *wanting* is not the same as *choosing*.

As I wrestled with this idea, I came across another helpful phrase they use that says, "When the struggle starts, get happy." It sounds counterintuitive, but it means this: conflict precedes clarity. If you are struggling, it means change is already in motion. You are not stuck—you are shifting. Transformation is happening.

I love how the Medicine Wheel teaches balance, not perfection. It acknowledges that pain and joy, loss and renewal, struggle and ease—all of these coexist. And if we allow ourselves to truly process all our experiences—to let them pass through us like that funnel in my dream— they refine us.

Looking back, I now see that every experience—even the worst ones— have contributed to my growth. Everything, when processed and healed, has the potential to transform us into something better. We are not just the sum of our parts. We are the alchemy of our experiences.

I miss our long conversations, the way we would lose track of time unraveling the mysteries of life. You always had a way of helping me see things from a new perspective, helping me through the refining process. If you were here, I know you'd have some profound insight that would likely add to everything I just wrote.

For now, I'll just imagine your knowing smile and send my love your way...

- *L*

39. *Seeing Clearly*

I had an appointment with the optometrist today, and guess what he found? Astigmatism.

Seriously? The poetic irony is both comical and tragic. I've already spent years struggling with the stigma of being an alcoholic and having a substance use disorder, and now I have astigmatism too?

Naturally, I had to look up the definitions.

Stigma: "A mark of disgrace associated with a particular circumstance, quality, or person." (Synonyms: shame, disgrace, dishonor, stain, taint, blot, blemish, brand, mark)

Astigmatism: "A defect of an optical system resulting in a blurred and imperfect image." Also described as: "Distorted understanding suggestive of the blurred vision of an astigmatic person."

How ironic. You know how much I have resented the stigma placed on both of us by others—their distorted, imperfect perception of what it means to be a sufferer of SUD (which gets reduced to the label "*alcoholic*"). And then, to find out that I, too, have astigmatism, a literal defect that distorts how I see things. I can almost hear you saying, "Mmm hmm."

It reminds me of that old verse about pointing out the speck in someone else's eye while ignoring the plank in your own. How often have I felt frustrated with how others see me, without questioning the distortions in my own vision? I realize now that I also distorted the information coming in from others in such a way that often bolstered either the shaming beliefs about myself, or my judging criticism of them.

It seems like most of the world has a form of astigmatism when it comes to understanding addiction—whether you're the sufferer or a bystander. Our perception is often blurred, clouded by misinformation, outdated beliefs, or an unwillingness to see beyond our own biases. Many of us have triggers and wounds from past experiences that also skew our outlook. Without better education, we assume addiction is just a lack of willpower, that it's a moral failing, that people who struggle with it are weak and selfish. We look at those in recovery with pity, embarrassment, or judgment.

But our vision is flawed; we don't see the whole picture. You know how I used to care so much about how others saw me. Even now, as I've grown more comfortable with my story, I still catch that flicker of discomfort in people's eyes when I mention my addiction. Some react with subtle pity, as if I need to be consoled. Others seem embarrassed for me, as though my truth is too raw for them to handle. It is as if they feel shame on my behalf, even when I don't feel it for myself so much anymore.

But their reaction isn't about me. It's about them. Their own astigmatism. And I no longer feel the need to own it.

The stigma surrounding substance use disorders seems to always find its root in the whole controversy around whether it is a disease or a choice. Having lived it firsthand, it never truly felt like a choice for us. We didn't wake up one day and decide, "You know what would be fun? Slowly destroying my life with alcohol." Instead, it was a long, seemingly unavoidable progression, almost imperceptible, until the manifesting symptoms were too significant to ignore.

Personally, it's hard for me to understand why some hesitate to call alcoholism a disease. After all, no one argues whether cancer or diabetes are diseases—so why does addiction still seem to be up for debate? Substance use disorder (SUD) is a medical condition, and if we could accept it as such, I believe the stigma would be reduced. But instead, it feels like the whole topic is still taboo—too often dismissed, judged, or ignored entirely.

I once heard Dr. McCauly argue, "If someone held a gun to your head and told you not to drink, you wouldn't." He claims substance addiction is a choice of volition, meaning it is internally generated. But then he goes on to explain that while, in theory, there is an element of choice, addiction hijacks the brain and disrupts common reasoning—making good decisions feel nearly impossible. These fundamental changes in neurological function are also what make stopping so incredibly difficult.

Reframing SUD as a disease helps reduce the stigma and remove the shame. In doing so, sufferers can move past the humiliation and judgment that have kept them from seeking help. It allows them to step out of the shadows and admit they need treatment—without the added weight of moral condemnation.

Understanding my own astigmatism and how I have misinterpreted other people's actions or responses to my drinking has also been helpful. It has allowed me to reframe the way distance sometimes becomes necessary when someone is in the depths of addiction. Just like certain illnesses require isolation to prevent further harm, addiction, too, can create situations where loved ones have to step back for their own well-being. I know that when I was drinking, my words and actions hurt people—sometimes deeply. And while boundaries were needed, what made all the difference was whether they were set with love and hope, or with judgment and shame. There's a fine line between creating space to protect oneself and using distance as a form of silent punishment. One offers a bridge back. The other builds a wall.

Alcoholism and drug addiction are among the few diseases where, all too often, the default response isn't compassion—it's anger, disgust, and blame.

I think of a woman I met in treatment named Sarah. She had been a highly respected nurse practitioner before drug use and alcoholism took over her life. By the time Sarah got to rehab, she had lost her medical license, her practice, and most of her relationships. But what haunted her most wasn't what she had lost—it was the way people now looked at her.

Sarah said that a few years back, when she told people she had breast cancer, they rallied around her. When she told people she had a substance use disorder, they recoiled. Some offered sympathy laced with judgment, others avoided her entirely.

Both were diseases. One was met with compassion. The other was met with disgrace.

That's what stigma does. It isolates people. It keeps them from getting help. It makes them believe they are beyond redemption.

Substance use disorder is treatable. If caught early enough, the body and brain can heal. But like any other disease, if left untreated, it can progress to a point of no return. And the stigma surrounding it often keeps people from seeking help until it's too late.

I have spent so many years of my life being ashamed of who I was, especially when I realized that I was addicted to alcohol—hiding, pretending, not wanting anyone to know my "dirty little secret." But now, I see things more clearly.

I understand that I did not make myself an alcoholic. Neither did you. We did not "contract" this disease because we were weak or because we lacked self-control. We were born with a predisposition, and in the case of alcoholism, the disease *is* the predisposition.

Research shows that two people can drink the same amount, and one will develop a dependency while the other won't—largely due to their unique biological responses. It's not about willpower or some personality defect. It's about how the brain and body interact with the substance. And, unfortunately, there's currently no way to know for certain what a given person's biological response will be before they take those drinks.

While I will take responsibility for the things I said and did while in my disease state, I refuse to carry shame for having the predisposition that caused my drinking to develop into the medical condition of substance use disorder. I accept that this disease is a part of my story. Maybe it was always going to be, as a part of some bigger plan. I don't know why. But I don't carry shame about that anymore.

If someone looks down on me, if they pity me, if they see me as blemished because of my struggle, I now see that it's their own astigmatism that is distorting their view—it's *not* a true reflection of who I am. And their vision problem is just that - theirs - and I no longer feel the need to correct it.

So, here's to seeing clearly, to breaking the stigma, and challenging the distorted lens through which addiction is so often viewed.

And while I wish I could be looking at you face to face, I'll have to settle for seeing you in my mind's eye for now. But know this—no distortion or blurred vision could ever change how much I miss you. As always, I'm sending my love.

- *L*

40. Bear? What Bear?

You'll never believe what happened on my hike today. Actually, knowing me, you probably will. Let's just say I may need to start planning ahead a little better...

I decided to take a morning hike by myself today. On my way up the mountain, I admired the aspens and other deciduous trees awash with yellow, amid the dark evergreens. I could hear the occasional rustling of millions of little round leaves and the splashing water of the creek beside the trail.

When I eventually began crossing that creek, I stepped on some unstable rocks, toppled, and nearly went down into the water. I caught myself just in time, one leg stretched out behind me, and my arms spread like uneven airplane wings. Then, just as I made it to the far bank, three women rounded a corner, laughing loudly and chatting in a way that wasn't typical for quiet mountain trails. After pleasant hellos and a few comments about the weather, one of the ladies turned to me and asked, "Are you hiking alone?"

When I said yes, she gave me a concerned look. "Do you have bear spray?" I shook my head. "Well, you should at least hum or sing while you hike," she advised. "That way, you won't startle a bear. Startling them is what makes them aggressive."

Oh. Bears. Right. That's a thing here in Montana.

A little while later, another hiker with two big dogs confirmed that bears were definitely active in the area. He told me a mother bear and her two cubs had been spotted down by the water just two days ago. "They're more aggressive this time of year," he warned. "They're preparing for hibernation. Next time, bring bear spray."

He shared that grizzlies had even been seen recently in this area.

Grizzlies.

I chuckled nervously to myself as I realized I hadn't even considered the possibility of coming across a bear—even though I was literally hiking *Bear Creek Trail*.

So, for the next hour, I had full-on choir practice with myself, humming, singing, and making noise as I walked. And as I did, I thought about how this whole situation mirrored my life—how I try to feel safe by trusting in my ability to predict threats and protect myself, while also trying to fully take in the beauty and joy around me. It's a constant challenge to keep fear from taking the driver's seat.

At one point, I stopped to take in Bear Creek Falls, watching the water cascade down the mountain. Off to the side, I noticed a large flat rock right next to the river. I thought to myself, "What a great spot for a bear to get into the water and fish." It's here in the woods, surrounded by miles of wilderness. A true bear paradise.

The thought again struck me: How had I not anticipated bears on a trail literally named after them? How many times throughout my life have I—with all my anxiety and threat-detection systems—found myself just *strolling through bear country without a clue?*

By now, you probably guessed where my reflections are headed next…Even this reminded me so much of my experience with alcoholism.

When I first started drinking, I never considered that I might become an alcoholic. Sure, I knew addiction ran in families, but I thought it had more to do with personality or upbringing. I figured the people who ended up alcoholics were the ones who acted like alcoholics—the ones who mirrored their parents' behavior, had a certain type of character, or made reckless choices. Since I didn't see myself like that, I never imagined I could develop the same condition. I mean, my dad and I were very different people, right?

I didn't yet realize that addiction has biological and neurological roots—a genetic predisposition mixed with environmental factors, trauma, and for me, complicated grief. Like walking through bear country without bear spray, I was moving through life with a genetic predisposition to alcoholism and had no idea.

It didn't help that our culture has for a long time normalized alcohol as a coping mechanism. When things fall apart, what do people do? They drink. You don't see much about what alcohol does to the brain or body in the media, only that it's the go-to fix for stress, heartbreak, or a bad day.

The problem with addiction is that it doesn't stay the same—it's a progressive disease. The only thing predictable about it is that it will always get worse. I remember my sponsor telling me, "Alcoholism takes no hostages. It won't be satisfied until it takes your life." That stuck with me.

At least I know bears don't actually want to hurt me. They'll only attack if they're startled or provoked. Addiction? It doesn't care. It will destroy everything in its path. In that sense, bears are far safer than alcohol.

I wish there were better ways to educate people about the science of substance use disorders. If more people understood how addiction works—especially those with a family history of it—maybe fewer lives would be lost.

Speaking of family, I think about my grandkids a lot when it comes to this. There's alcoholism on both sides of their family tree, which means they have a 50-60% chance of developing the disease if they drink at all. That number stuns me. If someone told me I had a 50% chance of crashing on a flight, I wouldn't get on the plane. But that level of risk is a reality for them.

I want them to know the truth—that this isn't just about willpower or character or upbringing. That it's likely their bodies will react to alcohol differently than their friends' bodies will. That once addiction is triggered by the substance, it takes over.

And while we're at it, I'd also like to remind them to bring bear spray if they ever hike Bear Creek Trail in late fall. Because while I managed to avoid any actual bear encounters today, I did see fresh bear scat on the trail. They were nearby, watching from somewhere.

Still, I fully enjoyed the hike—the crisp air, the golden aspens, the sound of the rushing creek. I just wish you'd been there with me—laughing, singing, and probably making up ridiculous bear songs along the way. That would have been even better than bear spray.

Gotta go now. I'm off to grab a pastry from Smith's Bakery as a post-hike treat—I think I'll have a bear claw.

Sending my love,

- *L*

41. Excitement or Fear?

This morning, as I sat with my coffee, I watched a huge flock of quail darting around the yard—scratching at the earth, pecking at food, constantly vying for the best spot. If one of them found something worth eating, the rest rushed over in a frenzy, like they were terrified they'd miss out.

It made me laugh because, at first glance, they looked like little balls of anxiety—panicked, desperate. But then I stopped myself.

What if they weren't frantic with fear but thrilled with excitement? Maybe, after a long night, they were just eager for breakfast. Maybe what I saw as chaos was actually pure joy.

It got me thinking about that plaque in my office—the one that says, "The only difference between fear and excitement is your attitude about it." I've always loved that saying. It's scientifically true. Fear and excitement trigger pretty much the same physiological response in the body: increased heart rate, shortness of breath, a surge of adrenaline. The only difference is how we interpret the situation.

I smiled as I thought back to all the times we chased that blurred line between fear and excitement. Roller coasters, wild e-bike rides, spontaneous road trips into the unknown. We were ready to blaze the trails and swing from the trees. We knew how to lean into the thrill of the moment, how to embrace the rush of possibility.

But somewhere along the way, as life got more challenging, we lost that perspective. Instead of anticipating new opportunities with excitement, we started dreading worst-case scenarios. Instead of riding the wave, we let it pull us under. Instead of flowing with the rush of possibility, we seemed to drown under the weight of inevitability. And we weren't alone.

If we surveyed people across the country, I bet the number one answer to the question, "How are you feeling today?" would be, "Stressed." It used to be that depression was the most common mental health disorder in the U.S. Now, it's anxiety. And not just in the clinical sense. Most of the world feels on edge. We all felt the extra stress and fear around Covid, and that hasn't yet come all the way back down. Climate change, natural disasters, economics, and politics—on top of everyone's personal challenges—intensify the feelings of panic. All this added energy seems to have impacted us to the point of collectively accepting chronic anxiety as the new normal.

And it's no surprise that anxiety is the number one reason people give for drinking or using drugs—including prescriptions. People are desperate to quiet the constant hum of unease, to feel some sense of control.

But what if we could shift our perspective? What if, instead of assuming the worst, we trained ourselves to see possibility? What if we could anticipate something *better* instead of dreading something *worse*?

This shift in mindset—from powerless to empowered—is something I used to encourage my clients to practice. When they struggled with feeling helpless, I'd challenge them to start adding two words to everything they did: "I choose."

- "I choose to get out of bed."
- "I choose to make coffee."
- "I choose to go to work."

It sounds ridiculous at first, but it reframes the narrative. It reminds us that life isn't just happening to us. We are active participants. Even in our moments of inaction, we are still making a choice.

This is especially true for those of us caught in the struggle of addiction. We might not be able to simply choose not to drink—not in the way people think, anyway. But we *can* choose to get help. And that choice? That's where everything begins.

I remember every excuse I had for why going to treatment wasn't possible. There was no time. My schedule was packed with clients, and I was my mother's primary caregiver. There was no money. My insurance didn't cover inpatient treatment, and we were already struggling financially. How could I justify the ginormous bill for something I wasn't even sure would work? And then there was the guilt of knowing my illness was costing my family yet again.But here's the truth: it was worth every penny. At the time,

144

I didn't think my life had that kind of value. Now, I see it so clearly. It wasn't just money spent on treatment; it was an investment. And it has paid off tenfold. Because of that choice, I got my life back—a *new and improved* version, no less.

Yes, it was terrifying. But on the other side of fear is freedom. At the time, I had no idea how much better life could be. I had no way of seeing the future version of me—the one who now wakes up *excited* for the day instead of *dreading* it. Now, I'm more financially stable than I ever was while drinking. My practice has grown, my creativity has flourished, and I've been able to pursue work that actually inspires me. I have more clarity, more energy, more purpose. And the biggest payoff? I am free. Free is exciting.

We both know how hard it is to swallow our pride, to push past the excuses, to admit we need help. But if we can't make that choice in the moment, then we need to be ready to reach out when the hangover hits. There is never a wrong time to take the right step toward recovery.

And here's the thing: on the other side of fear is excitement. I know this now. The same energy that once fueled my despair is now fueling my joy. Life is unpredictable—yes—but that also means anything is possible.

I know you would understand exactly what I mean. You've always known how to find the fun in life, even when things got messy. I wish we could laugh about it together right now.

Sending My Love,

- *L*

42. *Nothing and Everything*

I keep thinking about all the times we laughed about the power of a zero. "If only we could add a few more of these!" We marveled at how a zero, which represents nothing on its own, could hold immense power when placed in the right circumstances (like on a paycheck). Funny how something so empty could mean so much.

Lately, I've been reflecting on how we all work so hard to build something—to "make something of our lives"—whether we are climbing the ladder in a corporation, striving to make a private business thrive, or growing and shaping a family. We work so hard to build something bigger, better, or higher, and then, inevitably, something in life comes along and pulls out the bottom block in the tower, causing everything to come crashing down. We tell ourselves we are working toward stability, toward something lasting, yet it seems life itself is built on impermanence.

I had my own "zero moment" when I walked through the doors of rehab, throwing all the carefully stacked cards of my life into the air, unsure of where they'd land. I didn't know if I'd have a career to return to. My family relationships were strained, my marriage barely holding on, my body wrecked. I felt like I had lost everything. (True, I was one of the lucky ones. My losses, while devastating, were not as catastrophic as they could have been. But they were great enough that I truly had to start over, with pretty much everything.)

There is a quote by Hafiz that says, "Zero is where the real fun starts; there's too much counting everywhere else."

At first, that idea seemed absurd to me. What could be fun about losing everything? But as I started to rebuild after rehab, I realized there was something oddly liberating about being at zero. When there's nothing left to hold onto, suddenly everything is possible. Without the weight of expectations, I could begin to explore new ideas, paths, and possibilities I had never considered before. Zero wasn't just an ending—it was an opening.

We spend so much of our lives preparing for the future: securing finances, planning for health concerns, anticipating challenges. And while preparation has its place, it also keeps us tethered to illusions of control. The only moment we truly have is this one. Right now. Everything else is a projection, a guess, a story we tell ourselves about what might happen. In that way, we are always at a kind of zero. A blank slate. A space of exciting and beautiful potential.

The Greek philosopher Heraclitus of Ephesus said, "You can never bathe in the same river twice." Thich Nhat Hanh expands on this idea:

> The river is always flowing, so as soon as we climb out onto the bank, even if we turn right back around to climb into the water, the water has already changed. And even in that short space of time, our bodies have also changed, with cells dying and being born every second. Even our thoughts, perceptions, feelings, and state of mind are changing from one moment to the next. So, we cannot swim twice in the same river; nor can the river receive the same person twice.

In the fall, after the trees change through their brilliant colors, they drop their leaves, which are no longer needed for the coming winter. I think of that as I work to let go of things that no longer serve me or the highest good. When there are situations I want to change or completely let go of, I pray and trust and move into that change. When I want to be free from limiting thoughts or habits, I mindfully let them go and claim a sort of spiritual freedom and power.

Just as trees release the old leaves to make room for new ones, my release of unhelpful practices makes room for new experiences. This allows me the space to grow and manifest the desires of my heart. When I feel myself being drawn into regret or resentment of the past, I gently bring my mind back to this present moment. When I start worrying or having anxiety about the future, I practice doing the same thing. Being present and mindful, embracing the truth that this moment is the only moment I have any power in, helps me stay grounded and more at peace.

To me, this is all in the same vein as the concept of "less is more." That sometimes as we let things go, or as we step away from the rat race of expectations, responsibilities, and obligations that aren't in line with our value system, we are able to receive more because our hands aren't already full. They are free and available to receive. We can then take advantage of the opportunity to be receptive in ways we didn't even know, for things we didn't realize we needed.

I think of this when I catch myself longing for what was or worrying about what will be. Like the river, life is always moving. Nothing stays the same—not the water, not us, not the circumstances that once seemed so permanent. The trees shed their leaves without resistance, making space for something new. If nature can let go so gracefully, why do we hold on so tightly?

It's a paradox: the less we cling, the more we receive. We spend our lives filling our hands with things we think we need, yet it's only when we let go that we make room for what we truly desire. The moment we stop grasping, we find ourselves open, receptive, free. And suddenly, zero is not emptiness. It's pure potential.

So, here's to zero. To fresh starts. To *not* knowing and being okay with it. To the wild, wonderful space where real life happens.

Sending you my L 0 ve...

- *L*

43. *The Weight of Trust*

Remember how we would laugh and shake our heads, saying, "No way!" when someone in the movies would say, "Trust me..." I don't know about you, but I tend to immediately distrust anyone who says that in day-to-day life, as well. To me, those can be empty words that don't mean much. If you want me to trust you, I need to see proof in the form of actions. And if you've broken my trust, I'm going to need to see evidence that I can trust you for quite a while before I can fully rely on you again.

Recently, however, I had to wrestle with my own complicated feelings around trust when *I* am the one who has broken it and is now asking to be trusted again.

I struggled with a tense discomfort as I found myself unexpectedly identifying with convicted criminals whose retrials were being publicly covered by the media. Of course, I haven't committed murder or any other serious crime, but being an "addict" can often elicit the same kind of disdain from society. I also know what it feels like to be judged by just one label. It seems like everyone knows someone who was killed or injured by a drunk driver, or someone who suffered horrendous abuse at the hand of an addict under the influence. I've felt branded by each person's worst experience with an alcoholic—clumped into a group titled, "menaces to society." In some cases, that isn't entirely wrong, but, just as with many criminal trials, there is more to the story with addiction.

Did I ever tell you about the survey Johns Hopkins did in 2014? They asked people about their willingness to engage with individuals who have substance use disorders, and here's what they found:

- Most people didn't want them as neighbors, employees, or family members.
- A significant portion thought they shouldn't receive the same level of health insurance coverage.
- Over 30% of respondents believed that people with addiction could never fully recover or lead productive lives.

When I see these results, I think to myself, *not only do people not want to help, they also don't think we're worth helping. They don't even believe in the possibility of recovery.*

Yet, as I come back to the topic of trust, I understand the difficulty. When it comes to people who have committed serious crimes, I believe I would be able to forgive them of their offenses, if they were genuinely sorry and in reform. At the same time, I'm not sure I would be comfortable with them moving in "next door."

And on a personal level, I do realize that when the trust between an offender and a victim is broken, this is probably similar to how others I've loved might feel toward me. Maybe ready to forgive, but not ready to trust.

Sometimes, trust has to take a back seat. For example, did you know that highway patrolmen are taught to assume three out of ten drivers are driving under the influence at any given time, with those numbers even higher on holidays or around special events? (This statistic was shared with me before COVID, and data shows the numbers have gone up since then.) The problem is prevalent, and society does not have compassion for someone who has made the "bad choice" of driving under the influence. It is difficult for them to accept that the offender didn't have the right mind to make a "good choice."

Truly, I share in the anger and grief when someone loses their life or health to the poor choices of a drunk driver. However, because of my personal experience and acquired knowledge, I know the harm rippling out from one driver's actions is the result of a disease. I believe that, ultimately, these offenses are worthy of forgiveness. I also believe that it takes time to earn trust again after causing others so much pain.

Truth is, all of us, at one time or another, have done the wrong thing for the "right" (or at least understandable) reasons. Perhaps this is part of why we have such a difficult time trusting other. We know that we, too, have the ability to "choose wrongly."

Understandably, there are people who still have trouble trusting me after my years of addiction. It's always difficult to earn back trust once it has been broken. It always takes time. And in some cases, forgiveness is never extended. I could try to justify all my excuses (many of them even valid, in my opinion), but the bottom line is, my actions caused injury. Maybe not the kind you see with your eyes, but certainly ones you feel with your heart. Accepting this truth is hard. And to be honest, I can understand why it would be hard to trust me. Sometimes, I'm not sure I can trust myself. And I, too, have difficulty trusting others, because we all have this messy human condition and are bound to fail at one point or another.

So rather than staying caught in feelings of failure or doom, I will instead glean wisdom from it. In my acceptance that everyone has wounds and weaknesses—moments of making compromised choices—my intention is to better support and encourage sufferers of SUD, allowing and helping them to heal. I hope to encourage them with the words my mentor has reminded me of time and time again, "I have chosen wrongly, but I can choose again."

Thank you for always trusting and believing in me, even when I probably didn't deserve it! I miss you! Sending my love,

- *L*

44. *Blueprint of a Soul*

Well, I had another wild dream last night. And this one has been coming in episodes—like my subconscious decided to produce a limited series starring me as the frazzled protagonist.

In this dream, I was on a relentless mission to track down a strange machine, about the size of an old stereo speaker, but way more powerful. It wasn't a bomb, a government tracking device, or even some secret high-tech coffee maker (which actually sounds quite useful). No, this thing held every single detail about my existence: my personal history, my ancestral lineage, my medical vulnerabilities, my past mistakes, and even information I wasn't supposed to know yet about the future. It contained my Akashic records, the history of my soul. It was all there—raw, unfiltered, impossible to deny.

At first, I was fascinated. Who wouldn't be? I was chasing after it out of curiosity. Who wouldn't want to unlock the full history and see the blueprint of their soul—the hidden threads woven into their life? But soon, the dream shifted. It wasn't just about discovery anymore—it was about survival.

Because in this dream, there were people using these machines not to enlighten or heal, but to sort, label, and determine who was "worthy" and who wasn't. Those of us with genetic flaws, addiction histories, and mental health challenges were considered lesser. Disposable. There was a new kind of supremacy movement rising, and with it, a terrifying plan to "cleanse" society. A modern-day Holocaust, not based on race or religion, but on what was hidden within our DNA. Red

What started as fascination quickly turned to terror. I thought of something you and I have said countless times, "Knowledge is power." It was practically a mantra when I worked in the schools, reminding kids that understanding the world and ourselves gives us the tools to make better choices. But if we aren't careful, the power to help can twist into something else. We can become power mongers, control freaks—obsessed with being above, knowing more, and having control over others.

We tend to believe that more information is always better—that if we just had all the data, we could predict everything, control outcomes, eliminate risk. I used to think how great it would be if we could test for the predisposition to alcoholism or addiction, or if we could catch debilitating diseases early. And maybe, in some cases, it *would* be wonderful. But what if that information was used against us? What if people with inherent weaknesses—like a genetic link to addiction—were disqualified or rejected before they ever had a chance to prove themselves?

Just as women used to be denied jobs because they *might* get pregnant, people could be denied opportunities because their DNA *might* carry a risk of cancer, lupus, or early-onset Alzheimer's. Imagine employers, insurers, even potential life partners scanning someone's genetic blueprint like a résumé—filtering out those deemed "too flawed."

Here's the thing: none of us would be immune. No matter how healthy, how stable, how put-together someone seems, we all carry weaknesses. Some are just more visible than others. Maybe if we kept that in mind, we'd be less quick to judge those suffering from addiction, mental illness, or chronic disease. Maybe we'd be more willing to see the person first, instead of their condition.

That's why I think true healing isn't just about medical intervention—it's about compassion. It's why the way I was treated in rehab made all the difference. I wasn't shamed. I wasn't punished. I wasn't treated like someone who needed to be "fixed" or erased. Instead, I was given care, understanding, and tools to heal. True healing requires knowledge of the condition and recognition of the whole person beyond it. That is what put me back on my feet. That is what made me a contributor to society again. That is what gave me my voice back so I could help others.

So now, I find myself wondering—what if we all carried around machines that exposed every part of our story? Would it make us kinder? Would it better equip us for the challenges ahead? Or would we keep trying to separate the "worthy" from the "unworthy"?

Because let's be honest—none of us are flawless. We all carry invisible wounds, genetic roll-of-the-dice conditions, or histories we'd rather not have written. And maybe if we could truly see all of it in one another, we'd stop pretending that anyone is somehow "better" or "less than."

I guess what I'm saying is this: If we ever do get a machine like the one in my dream, I hope we use it wisely. Not to divide, but to connect. Not to discard, but to understand.

And if a creepy little machine ever tells you someone is genetically inferior, just unplug it and throw it in the nearest lake, okay? In the meantime, I'll keep working on embracing my beautifully flawed humanity—and yours.

Missing you today and sending my love,

- *L*

45. *The Disease Debate*

To disease or not to disease—that is the question!

I had an interesting conversation with a client today, and it got me fired up all over again about this whole debate. He knows he needs help, but he isn't ready to admit he's addicted to alcohol, because—like so many others—he sees that as admitting failure. I get it. I really do. But it also makes me want to throw my hands in the air (or maybe at the nearest wall).

So, naturally, I shared some of my passionate, fact-filled thoughts with him—which will probably sound like a familiar rant to you. But you know me, I'm an external processor. I know you, of all people, will relate to this, because we've walked the same path.

Forgive me for repeating myself, as I know I probably have in several letters, but some things deserve to be repeated. The emphasis needs to get through so changes can be made.

I let my client know—as I have tried to scream through the megaphone so many times—that the American Medical Association officially recognized alcoholism as a *disease* in 1956.

That's almost seventy years ago. And yet, here we are, still arguing about it. Still having to justify it. Still watching people—even professionals—struggle to treat it as a disease. Why?

Substance use disorder (SUD) meets every single clinical criterion for disease:

- Onset of specific symptoms
- Predictable progression (early, middle, late stages)
- Potential for treatment
- High risk of relapse
- Fatal if left untreated

And yet, people continue to resist.

What confuses things, of course, is that not everyone who drinks too much has the actual disease of alcoholism. That depends on the biological and neurological makeup of the drinker. That is partly why some people can drink excessively for a while, and then just stop, like quitting a bad habit. Those with the disease are almost never able to "just stop" and get sober on their own.

Even medical professionals who understand this distinction can find it challenging, because individuals struggling with addiction almost always lie about or misrepresent their usage, making it difficult for providers to determine the best course of action.

If you ask me, I think our society has a hard time accepting SUD as a disease for three key reasons:

1. *People with the disorder don't want to admit they have a disease,* especially one that carries so much stigma and shame. For many, saying "I have an addiction" feels the same as saying "I'm weak" or "I'm a failure." And let's be honest—rational thinking isn't exactly at its peak when someone is deep in addiction. It's a disease that tells you that you don't have a disease.
2. *People without the disorder don't want to believe addiction is a disease* because they think it lets those with addictions off the hook. As if saying "it's a disease" means there's no accountability for one's own actions or the harm they've caused. Maybe there's even an underlying fear that if we recognize it as a legitimate medical condition, people will just keep drinking, using, and behaving recklessly without consequence.
3. *Most people—including medical and mental health professionals— just don't know what to do with someone suffering from addiction.*

That last one is huge.

Most doctors and therapists receive shockingly little education on addiction. Even trained professionals are often uncomfortable, unsure, or avoidant when faced with a patient struggling with it. Instead of treating SUD like other chronic illnesses, it gets pushed into the realm of "somebody else's problem." Patients are often dismissed, criminalized, or simply avoided.

This is why so many people suffering from addiction end up in the wrong places for help—prisons, detox centers with no follow-up care, hospitals that discharge them with no adequate plan, or therapy offices where the provider isn't trained in addiction at all. And this lack of training and preparation just reinforces the stigma. If the very people meant to help aren't comfortable dealing with it, how can we expect society at large to be?

I've shared in other letters how studies have been done that reveal people don't want to get involved with someone struggling with a substance use disorder. Too many people out there—professionals and non-professionals alike—are skeptical about the possibility of recovery. I believe a primary reason for this is because they don't accept it as a treatable disease.

And that's the sting of stigma.

The book *Understanding Addiction* sums it up perfectly:

> If we could get past these roadblocks around calling substance use disorder a disease, afflicted people would be able to receive proper medical treatment covered by health insurance. Not defining it as a disease means these people will be denied access to the right medical care. Considering SUD as a mere psychological disorder or worse, a moral failure instead of a disease means more people in prison and an unrelenting stigma that will keep them from seeking the help they need.

And yet, while acknowledging SUD as a disease is an important first step, it does not capture the full complexity of the issue. Dr. Gabor Maté has said that to simply call addiction a disease is too shallow. I understand that, too, because substance use disorder doesn't exist solely in the body. It arises from the whole person—from pain, trauma, disconnection, biology, and unmet needs. In that way, it shares something in common with many other chronic diseases, which rarely exist in isolation. Most serious medical conditions—whether diabetes, heart disease, or autoimmune disorders—impact multiple areas of a person's life. With SUD, that complexity is often amplified. It not only affects the body, but deeply entangles the mental, emotional, relational, and spiritual dimensions of a person's being.

The conclusion for me is that it *is* a disease—and also more than that. It's a disease with depth. One that requires a whole-person response. And that's why simply treating the symptoms isn't enough. It's a crucial start, but healing has to happen at every level.

It's not just a philosophical question. It's not just a debate for doctors, therapists, or researchers. (And in my opinion, those who still think it's a matter of professional *opinion* are actually causing harm.) The refusal to treat SUD as a disease directly impacts access to treatment. It determines whether people receive medical intervention or are left to suffer. Whether they find recovery or end up incarcerated.

Even after years of sobriety, I still feel the weight of stigma. I still sense that quiet judgment, the lingering doubt about whether people like me are *really* trustworthy, *really* capable, *really* healed.

For decades, society has been told that people with addiction are weak and selfish. That they just make bad choices, want a high or a crutch, and lack willpower—that they are psychologically and fundamentally flawed. But I want to change that.

Because here's what I know firsthand: *Recovery is possible. People with addiction can and do rebuild their lives. Those who seek treatment deserve medical care—not punishment. We are not less than. We can be trustworthy, and we can rebuild what is broken.*

I want people to understand that treating addiction as a disease is not about giving sufferers an easy way out. It's about giving them a way through.

The truth is, recovery does come with conditions—just like managing diabetes, heart disease, or any other chronic illness. And just like those illnesses, it requires the right treatment, the right support system, and lifelong care.
We can recover. We do recover. But first, people have to believe we can.

Thank you for always believing in me. I miss you!

Sending my love,

- *L*

46. Love Moves

Remember how annoyed we used to feel, shaking our heads and rolling our eyes whenever someone would flippantly say, "I'll pray for you," in that vague, well-meaning-but-actually-avoidant kind of way? It's like the spiritual equivalent of posting a "prayer hands" emoji on social media after a tragedy. A way to claim credit for acknowledging discomfort without actually engaging with it.

Now, don't get me wrong. I believe in prayer. I believe in sending love, in holding people with intention, and trusting in forces greater than ourselves. But I also believe in putting action behind our words. In doing something when we *can* and learning when we *can't*. Because if all we ever do is *think* about the suffering around us, without ever *engaging*, we're not helping. We're just avoiding.

And avoidance, as I've learned (mostly the hard way), is one of the most dangerous habits we can develop.

This comes to mind every time I drive through the city—when I see someone holding a cardboard sign at a stoplight, or catch a glimpse of people tucked beneath bridges in sleeping bags, or notice the quiet desperation of those pacing outside liquor stores, waiting for them to open their doors. I feel that pull—the one that says *do something*—but I also feel the instinct to look away. Because looking means *seeing*. And seeing means *caring*. And caring means *responsibility*.

Responsibility? That's a heavy weight.

So, most people—myself included, more times than I'd like to admit—choose the easy route. We say things to ourselves like, *I'm sure it will all work out*. Or *I'll pray for them*. We remove ourselves from the equation, reassure ourselves that it's not our problem, and move on.

Because here's the thing: fear tells us to step back. *Love* tells us to step forward. Most people think the opposite of fear is courage. But I believe the opposite of fear is *love*.

Love isn't passive. Love *moves*. Love shows up. Love doesn't just acknowledge suffering from a distance—it *engages* with it. That doesn't mean we all need to run out and personally rescue every person struggling with addiction. (God knows that doesn't work, especially when someone isn't ready to be helped.) But it does mean we can stop pretending we're powerless.

Because we *do* have power.

We can educate ourselves. If we love someone with a substance use disorder, we can attend Al-Anon or similar programs to learn how to take care of ourselves while engaging with them in a healthier way. We can break free from codependent behaviors and stop enabling cycles of destruction. We can learn how to set boundaries, how to safely and productively interact with those who struggle, and how to shift our own perspective so that we no longer see them as lost causes, but as people in pain.

As my mentor always says, "All behavior is either an extension of love, or a cry for love." If we could see addiction through that lens—not as a moral failing or a lack of willpower, but as a deep, unmet need—how differently would we show up? How differently would we treat the people we've written off as hopeless? How differently would we advocate for policies, for treatment, for education? How differently would we love?

Of course, I also know that there are times when we truly *can't* do anything other than pray and send loving energy. When we don't have the ability, the proximity, or the right timing to step in and all we can do is trust in something bigger than ourselves. This is where I lean into faith—the faith that God can hold others when I can't. That there's a bigger plan at work. I just think we need to be careful not to let fear convince us we are powerless when we are not.

I think of people I care about who live far away, including you, dear friend, and how sending my love is still a genuine act. And I'll strive to take the opportunity when it arises to make even the smallest gesture—a handwritten note, a phone call, a bouquet of flowers—to remind someone they aren't forgotten. That their pain has been seen. That their life *matters*.

So yes, I will pray. But I will also *do*.

And I believe wherever you find yourself, you will, too.

Missing you and sending my love,

- *L*

47. *Perfect Timing*

I just heard another great quote attributed to Albert Einstein: "The reason for time is so all things don't happen at once." Naturally, that sent the Chicago song playing in my head—"Does anybody really know what time it is?"

I don't know about you, but my relationship with time is...complicated. Every morning, before I even get out of bed, I instinctively check the clock—like a contestant in *The Amazing Race*, trying to gauge whether I'm ahead or already impossibly behind. Will I have time to enjoy my coffee, or am I running late before the day even begins? I find myself doing mental gymnastics right out the gate—calculating how much time I have, what I need to get done, and how I can somehow manipulate the clock to stretch time in my favor.

And I know I'm not alone. The whole world seems to operate under an invisible stopwatch, demanding we rush through everything—work, meals, conversations, even relaxation. Productivity is worshiped, efficiency is expected, and patience? Well, patience is for people who *clearly* don't have as much to do as the rest of us.

I've been thinking about how much time I've spent worrying about time. I've hurried through conversations, already thinking of the next task. I've rushed through experiences, focused on what's *next* instead of what's *now*. And I realize how much impatience has stolen from me.

Truth be told—and I'm sure this is no surprise to you by now—patience has always been a challenge for me. I've always been a mover and a shaker— someone who likes to *make* things happen. But I've learned (mostly the hard way) that forcing things before their time rarely leads to good results.

Impatience keeps me from being fully present with myself, with others, and with life itself. When I'm impatient, I'm not *with* someone; I'm pushing them, or waiting for them to catch up to wherever I think we *should* be. And I think this is one of the ways impatience can feel unkind, even unloving. It doesn't take the time to meet the other person where they are to create a beautiful experience together. It tries to force something instead of letting it develop.

I see this in so many ways. In the way I want people to heal faster than they're ready to. In the way I get restless in long conversations, wanting to jump to the

point or the resolution. In the way I sometimes expect myself to be further along in my own healing than I actually am.

I believe this was yet another reason why I drank. Alcohol was my way of trying to reject time. It let me fast-forward through pain, mute emotions I wasn't ready to process, and hit pause on whatever reality I didn't want to face. Sobriety, on the other hand, has been about learning to *trust* time. To sit in discomfort, knowing it will pass. To wait for healing, believing it will come. To believe, despite my impatience, that things are unfolding exactly as they should.

Of course, that doesn't mean I *like* waiting. I still have that restless part of me that wants to see immediate results. But I've started noticing how, when I stop trying so hard to control the timing of things, they often have a way of falling into place.

Take rehab, for example. I was *not* on board with the timing of that. I had clients, responsibilities, a mother in hospice, financial pressures. Everything in me screamed that it was the wrong time to step away from my life. And yet, looking back, I can see it was the only time I *could* have done it. If I had waited until things "settled down," I wouldn't have made it. That timing was perfect—I just couldn't see it at the time.

It makes me think of the barn cat I often watch, crouched perfectly still in the grass, waiting for the right moment. Not anxious. Not second-guessing. Just *waiting*, fully present, trusting the moment will come for it to go after its prey. I envy that kind of patience.

If I really think about it, the universe has been incredibly kind in its gift of time. The lessons I've needed, the healing I've longed for, the relationships I've cherished—they haven't always arrived when I *thought* they should, but they've all arrived exactly when they were supposed to.. Looking back, I can see how moments of waiting—even the frustrating ones—were preparing me for something better than I could have imagined.

I think about my struggle with addiction and how, for years, I was impatient with myself. I wanted to be better *instantly*, to prove to myself and others that I had everything under control. But healing doesn't work that way. Just like a flower doesn't bloom before it's ready, true transformation happens on its own timeline. It can't be rushed, no matter how much we wish it could be. There is an Italian proverb that says, "The salt of patience seasons everything."

These days, I'm working on trusting that things will unfold as they should—that the conversations I need to have, the work I need to do, and the dreams I want to chase will all come together in their perfect time. And while I'd love to speed things up when they feel too slow, I also don't want to miss what's happening right now.

Truth be told, I'm not happy about the timing of our being apart. I really miss you, my friend, but I will try to trust that all is as it needs to be.

Impatiently—I mean, in patience—sending my love.

- *L*

48. From HALT to HOPE

Did you ever learn the acronym **HALT**? It stands for *Hungry, Angry, Lonely, and Tired*—four powerful triggers that can send someone spiraling into cravings for alcohol or other substances. I learned about them in rehab, and let me tell you, every single one of them played a role in my drinking.

Take hunger, for example. There were so many times I felt an urgent need to drink, but when I paused to check in with myself, I realized I was just hungry. My body, completely out of sync after years of drinking, confused signals of hunger with anxiety, which I reflexively tried to fix with alcohol. The irony, of course, is that alcohol never *fixes* anything. It just pushes the real problem further down the line.

Anger? Oh, mine wasn't the kind that exploded outward—it was more of an internal agitation, an ongoing frustration with all the ways my life wasn't what I wanted it to be. But I didn't *feel* angry. I just felt…stuck. Worn down. Depressed. And what better way to numb that vague yet overwhelming dissatisfaction than to pour a drink and let it blur into the background?

Loneliness, though—loneliness was the one that had its grip on me the longest. You already know how socially awkward I can be. You've known me long enough to have gotten used to it, which is probably why I miss you so much these days! I've always carried a certain discomfort in social situations. I can show up, present well, even enjoy myself sometimes—but underneath, I've spent my whole life feeling like an outsider.

I still cringe when I remember how, as a kid, my dad would make comments about how I might be "socially retarded" (his words, not mine). I was shy, insecure, and had a hard time making and keeping friends. I had people around me, sure, but I often felt like a placeholder—someone people invited because I had a pool, or because I was an easy second choice for companionship if no better option came along.

Over time, I learned how to "people-please" my way into acceptance. I figured out what others wanted me to be and adjusted accordingly. It worked—I was liked, included. I just had to make sure I didn't accidentally let my real self show, with all its quirks and blunders.

Loneliness is a strange thing. So many people who struggle with addiction are socially anxious or feel like they don't quite fit in. Drinking or using drugs helps them "loosen up" so they can *finally* be themselves—or at least the version of themselves they *want* to be. But here's the kicker: drinking to ease loneliness only guarantees deeper loneliness. It builds invisible walls instead of bridges, creating a cycle that ensures real connection will always stay just out of reach.

And then there's the *T*—Tired. Insomnia had been my constant companion long before alcohol entered the picture, but by my forties and fifties, it had become downright unbearable. Drinking seemed like a solution, and it kind of worked for a while. But even though alcohol helped me *fall* asleep, it never let me *stay* asleep. I'd wake up in the middle of the night, wired from the sugar in the alcohol, which kicked my racing thoughts into overdrive and made it impossible to drift off again. Multiple sleepless nights bred a growing fear—an anxious anticipation of the insomnia itself—which led to drinking the next night. And the next. The vicious cycle continued, leaving me more exhausted, more drained, and more desperate for an escape.

Even now, in recovery, I keep an eye on these triggers. I know relapse is always a possibility. If I find the thought or desire to drink creeping in, I check the HALT symptoms. I make sure I eat. I acknowledge and process my emotions. I reach out when I feel isolated. And I prioritize rest, knowing that exhaustion makes everything else harder.

But the story doesn't end with HALT and thankfully, neither did mine.

In rehab, I learned another acronym: **HOPE.**

Hold On, Pain Ends.

It doesn't promise an escape. It doesn't offer a magical solution. It simply reminds us that whatever we're feeling—no matter how unbearable it seems—it is temporary. The storm won't last forever. The sun is still shining behind the clouds, waiting for its moment to break through.

Recovery has taught me how to sit in discomfort instead of scrambling for immediate relief. This, in turn, has strengthened my resilience, just like exercise strengthens muscles by first tearing them down. It's helped me to surrender my need for control and to trust the process.

The storms *do* pass. And often, they leave behind a rainbow—a beautiful, unexpected reminder that there's still magic and hope on the other side. I love rainbows.

Thank you, dear friend, for always accepting me, awkwardness and all. I miss you. I wish I could discuss all of this in person, over coffee, while watching the world go by. For now, I'll just imagine my favorite rainbow arching over you.

Sending my love,

- *L*

49. The Gift of Wonder

Have you ever just watched a spider descending from above, creating its own lifeline as it goes? It's quite amazing if you think about it. The spider secretes a single strand—strong enough to support its body weight against the wind, yet so delicate that we can barely see it. How does it know the silk will hold? How does it trust something it's spinning in real time?

Miracles like these keep me fascinated. And I came by it honestly.

My mother had a gift for wonder. I remember how she would look up at the clouds, with no less enthusiasm than the day before, and say, *"I've never seen anything like that before!"* She would see an ordinary tree or flower and marvel at its beauty as though it were the first time she had ever laid eyes on such a thing. Even when her heart was heavy with life's burdens, she found delight in the smallest, simplest moments. She was an expert at curiosity and appreciation.

Some of the wisest advice I've ever received is to *just be curious*. When I would be frustrated with my own feelings, behaviors, or choices, my mentor would gently say, *"Be curious about that."* Not judgmental. Not anxious. Not dismissive. And that simple shift changed everything.

As a therapist, I am often curious about what's going on with my clients as they tell me about their situations and challenges. I enjoy being curious about the possible solutions that might help them. Keeping an attitude of curiosity, wonder, and delight allows us to find some enjoyment, even when parts of a situation feel hard. If we choose to evaluate ourselves and the circumstances we're in with openness and receptivity, better solutions will often come our way.

As I began my journey in sobriety, my curiosity was all about addiction itself. *Why did I end up with substance use disorder? What was it inside me that took me to that place?* I became fascinated by other people's stories— those who ended up in the same boat. Their backgrounds were wildly different, yet somehow, we all arrived at the same destination. At some point, my curiosity shifted from the kind that needs solutions to the kind that embraced the process. Do you know what I mean?

I started asking different questions. *How can I grow through this? What brings me joy? What would make me feel alive again?*

Curiosity became an anchor in my healing. It kept me open, even when I didn't have solutions. I didn't need to have everything figured out—just a willingness to explore, to wonder, to see what happened next.

Being curious has allowed me to remain open, like my mother did, to explore ideas and possibilities without becoming too attached to the outcome. When I stay in that attitude of wonder, I get to look at things from several different perspectives, maybe as a scientist or philosopher would, but without needing to define it. It's like looking at a difficult topic as an open-ended question or dialogue rather than a statement of fact.

Honestly, curiosity has saved me in more ways than one. I've found that being curious is a wonderful antidote to judgment and defensiveness—especially in conversations where I might otherwise struggle to relate. I recently had an interaction with a young adult client who was telling me about their love for dark, scary video games. Now, this is *not* my world. If I had to choose between playing a horror game and, say, cleaning out the fridge, I'd probably still choose the fridge.

But instead of dismissing it, I got curious. I listened. I asked questions. And what I learned was incredible. This client wasn't just playing games for entertainment—they found relief, challenge, even a sense of control in those virtual worlds. It was something that gave them joy. Something that helped.

If I had brushed it off as unimportant simply because it didn't resonate with me, I would have missed the opportunity to understand them better. And in that understanding came appreciation. Isn't that an important component of loving or connecting with someone else? The willingness to lean in, to listen, to be open?

I smile as I think of a young child exploring their surroundings. Everything is exciting and new. They don't have an attitude of "I know." In fact, they have the delight of not knowing and not needing to know, as far as facts go. They are truly caught up in the amazement of the moment—watching an interesting new bug, a soaring bird, a puddle that ripples just so. Their world is wide open, limitless in possibility. I want to be like that!

It brings to mind a challenge one of my mentors gave to the group at a recent training. At the beginning of class, she told us to avoid ever saying "I know." Because the moment we say that, we close the door to learning. We shut out new information and let our egos take control. We block the chance to expand, to discover something deeper, something more.

I think about how often we try to fit things into neat, understandable boxes. But life is so much bigger! Miracles are everywhere. Questions and curiosities are endless. And when we stop needing to *know* all the answers, we can finally dance and flow with the wonderment of our lives instead of trying to contain it.

John O'Donohue said,

> Wonder is a beautiful style of perception; when you wonder at something, your mind voyages deep into its possibility and nature. Wonder enlarges the heart. When you wonder, you are drawn out of yourself. The cage of ego and the rail tracks of purpose no longer hold you prisoner. Wonder is such a tiny word; yet it confers the highest dignity and mystery.

Right now, I'm wondering what you're up to. And I wish you were here to wonder with me. I miss you, and as always, sending my love.

- *L*

50. More Than a Word

Remember all the times we laughed at how ridiculous the word "love" is? How absurd it is that we use the same word for loving a sandwich as we do for loving a child? Or how we can love a good vacation and love a dying friend? At least the Greeks tried to sort it out, giving us *eros* (romantic love), *philia* (friendship love), *storge* (familial love), *mania* (obsessive love), and *agape* (selfless, unconditional love). But even that doesn't fully capture love's complexities. Love isn't static—it shifts, bends, and evolves with each new situation. It's the most powerful force we experience, yet we throw the word around so casually, applying it to everything from a favorite coffee to the deepest connections of our souls.

Add to that the understanding that love is more than just an emotion. It is also a myriad of actions. Maybe that's why love can be so hard to recognize when it arrives, because love doesn't always look, feel, or act the way we expect it to.

Sometimes, love is easy—warm hugs, laughter at the dinner table, hands held in hospital rooms, and long talks with a friend who just *gets* you. Other times, love is painful. It's a friend telling you something you don't want to hear. It's a boundary being set. It's a heartbreaking decision made in the best interest of someone else. Love doesn't always show up wrapped in comfort; sometimes it arrives in the cloak of disappointment, frustration, even loss. Love has many faces.

I think about the ways people loved me when I was struggling with my addiction. Some of them were obvious—people who sat with me, held my hand, cried with me, and told me they wanted me to get better. But there were also ways people loved me that I didn't recognize at the time.

There was my therapist, who—after listening patiently for months—finally told me, *"You need inpatient treatment. You don't just need help. You need a whole system of help."* At the time, I felt defensive, embarrassed. But looking back, I know that was one of the truest acts of love I've ever received. There was my daughter, who pleaded with me to get help, her eyes filled with tears as she told me she had dreams of me dying from this disease. There was my son and daughter-in-law, who—out of love—set firm boundaries, making it clear that, while they wanted me in their lives, I would not be allowed to care for my grandchildren if I was still drinking. And then there was my husband, who, in my lowest moments, simply said: "*I believe in you.*"

It didn't always feel like love at the time. Some of it felt like rejection. Some of it felt like judgment. Some of it felt like loss. But now, from the other side, I see it for what it was. Love doesn't always feel good, but it always tells the truth. And truth, at times, results in boundaries.

I now understand that even stepping away can be an act of love. When someone is in the throes of addiction, creating space can be necessary—not out of punishment, but out of protection. Just like we isolate during contagious illness to avoid further harm, substance use disorder can call for distance to safeguard the emotional and mental well-being of others. I know that during my drinking, my words and actions caused pain— sometimes lasting wounds. The boundaries people set were essential, but what truly impacted me was the spirit in which they were set: when rooted in compassion and hope, they opened the door to healing; when driven by judgment or rejection, they only deepened the shame.

This is a fine line to walk. Too often, people misuse the concept of *tough love*, twisting it into an excuse for excommunication. I see it happen all the time with addiction. Families or communities cut people off, saying, "They have to hit rock bottom. We have to teach them a lesson." And while boundaries are necessary, abandonment is not love. Shame is not love. Love does not exile. True love holds space for people while protecting itself as appropriate. It doesn't enable, but it also doesn't condemn.

What further complicates our understanding of love is the fact that love looks different to each person. Years ago, when our young family was in crisis, we created a family motto that included the word *respect*. But the funny thing was, each of us had a different idea of what that word meant. For one of us, respect meant not yelling. For another, it meant being patient. For another, it was listening with engagement. It made me realize that we throw around big words—love, respect, trust—without ever asking what they actually mean to the person standing in front of us.

Love will look different to each of us, depending on our needs and experiences. It will call us to act in ways that might not make sense to someone else. It might look like patience. It might look like truth. It might look like staying. It might look like leaving. But the one thing love *never* looks like is indifference. You and I have talked often about how the opposite of fear is love. But what about the antagonist of love? It's not hate, as many might assume. The opposite of love is indifference.

I've been thinking about this a lot lately. The truth is, I don't want to be talking about addiction. I don't want this to be my story. I would rather tuck it away, move on, and never bring it up again. While I'd never say I am indifferent to the subject, I would be happy to quietly ignore it. Sometimes I tell myself staying quiet protects other people—that no one really wants to hear about alcoholism and recovery, and that I should keep it to myself to avoid making others uncomfortable. But the reality is that, when I'm silent about it, the one I'm actually protecting is myself. Because I don't want to be defined by this. I don't want people's eyes to shift when I mention it, their expressions to tighten as they try to figure out if I'm one of *those* people. I don't want to be seen as weak or broken. I don't want the judgment or the assumptions. I want to keep moving, to focus on something else—anything else. And yet…I can't.

Because knowing what I know—both the science and the lived experience—how can I do nothing? People are dying. Lives are being destroyed. And it's not because people are inherently bad—it's because they don't know any better. Let's state, for the record, what you and I know to be true: Addiction is a war on love. You and I have always said that if you want to conquer something, you have to take away its power source. And what is the power source of love? Connection.

Now think about addiction. What does it do? It numbs. It isolates. It disconnects. Anyone who has struggled with a substance use disorder will tell you that they drank or used to escape something—to avoid pain, to avoid relationships in their messiness, to avoid themselves. If I were the enemy of love, what better weapon could I create than a substance that makes people stop *feeling*? I'd craft something that dulls the longing for connection, that dims vibrant souls into mere shadows of themselves.

Addiction doesn't just destroy individuals—it destroys families, communities, and entire generations.

As much as I don't want to deal with this, as much as I would rather look away, I *cannot do nothing* when I see this problem growing exponentially. Love can only win when we allow it to be a participant.

If the people around me had chosen indifference—if my family, my friends, my community, and the rehab staff had all looked the other way—I don't believe I would be sober today. In fact, it's more than likely I would not even be alive today. But love stepped in. It looked different from different people. For some, it was boundaries. For some, it was honesty. For some, it was a steady, unwavering belief in me. But love—in all its forms—is what saved me.

So now, I have to ask myself: what does love require of *me*? I believe love is the most powerful force in existence. To speak the love language of those who cross my path—whether they are struggling with addiction themselves, in relationship with someone who is, or simply trying to navigate their own life—I need to meet them where they are. So I've found these questions to be a great place to start: *What does love look like to you in this moment? What do you need? What do you desire? What can you do to facilitate or be open to love?*

I also like to remind people that the love we need often comes from within ourselves (if we allow it) as much as it comes from others. Self-love brings out some of our best qualities: respect, patience, self-discipline, gratitude, and humility. It is a key component for each of us, and it is crucial for successful recovery. What's more, the love we give others will be enhanced by the love we give ourselves.

Most things in life come and go, but love remains. It is our core, our essence, our connection to the divine. When we act in love—whether giving or receiving, we are aligning with our truest nature. I think of this quote by Talia Hunter that has been so helpful to me during my recovery.

> Anything that is not love is only a visitor to your body.
> You are not anxious, stress is simply flowing through you.
> You are not permanently depressed, sadness is simply visiting you.

You are not lost, confusion is simply wandering within you.
And you are not broken, pain is simply passing through you.

As I remain open to love, in whatever way it calls, I smile, and I think of it the way Ram Daas says, "We're all just walking each other home."

So, dear friend, know that I'm here and thinking of you. I wish you were closer, but just as love is big enough to transcend past, present, and future, I trust it's big enough to span the space between us.

I miss you, and I *philia* you. Always.

- *L*

51. *Dying in Plain Sight*

I need to vent. And right now, you're the only one I can do this with. So, here we go.

I've been looking at the latest statistics around addiction, and honestly? I feel sick. I feel scared. I feel *angry*. And I don't know what to do with all of it.

We are in the middle of the worst addiction crisis this country has ever seen, yet we're still acting like it's not a full-blown public health emergency. The numbers don't lie—people are *dying* at rates we've never seen before. And what are we doing about it? Not nearly enough.

Did you know that overdoses are now the number one cause of accidental and preventable death in the U.S.? Not car accidents. Not suicides. Not gun violence. Drug overdoses. According to the CDC, there were over 107,000 drug-related deaths in 2023 alone.

To put that in perspective, that's like a fully packed football stadium of people disappearing every year. Gone. Can you imagine how many surviving loved ones that impacts?

And then there's alcohol, specifically. It's a silent killer and we're not talking about it enough. Because while other drugs are fast and brutal, alcohol is quietly killing people at a staggering rate.

Alcohol-related deaths increased by 43% from 2006 to 2018—and have continued rising. In 2023, nearly 29 million people met the criteria for alcohol use disorder (AUD), but most never got treatment. 140,000 Americans die every year from alcohol-related causes. That's **one person every four minutes.** One in three liver transplants in the U.S. is due to alcohol-related liver disease.

And yet, alcohol still gets a free pass in our culture. It's *celebrated*, marketed at every turn, pushed at every social event. The message is clear: drink up. It's fun. It's normal. It's fine. Until it's not.

This isn't just a problem—it's a medical crisis.

While addiction is not just a mental health disorder (as it was believed to be for centuries), it does often coexist with one. Again, the numbers are staggering:

- Over 45% of people with SUD also have a co-occurring mental health condition, such as depression, anxiety, PTSD, or bipolar disorder.
- Many of them are trying to self-medicate without realizing that substances will ultimately make their conditions worse.
- ***People with SUD are six times more likely to die by suicide*** than the general population.

And yet, as a society, we still approach these issues separately when we should be tackling them together. Look at these statistics for 2023 alone:

- 49 million people aged 12 or older had a substance use disorder.
- That's 17.1% of the U.S. population—one in every six people you know.

This includes nearly 28.9 million people with alcohol use disorder,27.2 million people with a drug use disorder, and 7.5 million people with both.

WWWWHHHHHAAAAATTTT??? This is not a footnote—it's a title page. It doesn't call for band-aids—it calls for a crash cart!

How can we just sit around and wait until 17% of the people we love become overdose statistics? This is an active, growing problem that needs attention NOW.

There is so much more that I can't fully address in this letter—like how it's not just a numbers game; it's a matter of justice. There are real racial disparities in both treatment and death rates. This epidemic is hitting Black, Latino, and Indigenous communities at *higher rates* than other populations, with the death toll rising—yet these communities have the least access to medical care and treatment options. Systemic barriers—fewer healthcare providers, limited treatment facilities, racial prejudice in medicine—are making it even harder for people to get help before it's too late.

Did you know that less than five percent of people who need treatment for a substance use disorder ever receive it? Even the lucky few who get help often don't receive evidence-based care. Sixty percent of residential treatment facilities don't offer any addiction medication, and only *one percent* of all facilities offer all three FDA-approved medications for opioid use disorder.

While I was in rehab, I was given Naltrexone, Gabapentin, and Clonidine. These medications helped *tremendously* with cravings and withdrawal symptoms. While I tapered off everything else before leaving the treatment center, I continued taking Naltrexone for a few more months to stabilize my recovery. These medications weren't mood-altering. They weren't addictive. They simply made recovery more manageable.

You probably know as well as I do that most people can't access these life-saving medications because ***insurance won't cover them.*** Only sixty percent of employer-sponsored health plans even cover addiction treatment, and when they do, it tends to be quite limited. Additionally, insurance companies require prior authorization, delaying treatment when people are at their most vulnerable.

Imagine if only five percent of people with cancer got treatment. Imagine if insurance companies decided diabetes wasn't worth covering. The outrage would be instant. But because it's addiction—something we might wrongly label "bad choices"—we keep looking the other way. We've got to stop choosing to put our heads in the sand. We need to quit believing it's hopeless or brushing it away like it is someone else's problem.

Maybe because it is so poorly covered, or maybe because it's so poorly understood, physicians and medical professionals are NOT being adequately trained to understand and treat addiction. In a recent survey of physicians and nurse practitioners, only one in four said they'd received *any* addiction training during medical school. Even those who *did* said the training was extremely limited. Why is that? And why, if they didn't receive the training in medical school, have they not sought additional training outside of school?

We need to make some noise. We need to create change. We need to educate ourselves and others. We need an effective strategy to counter this epidemic before millions more die.

The knowledge is there for the gaining. The solutions exist. It just requires effort.

I so wish you were here to join me on this crusade. I don't know how much of this you knew before you left. I just wish I could hear your thoughts; hear you tell me it's going to be okay.

But since I can't, I'll settle for hoping you can still hear me somehow.

Sending my love, always.

- *L*

52. *The Empty Chair*

One year.

One whole year, today, without you.

I don't even know what to do with that reality. I still catch myself reaching for my phone, wanting to send you a message. There are things I need to tell you. Things I wish we could still talk about. But instead, I'm sitting here, staring at this empty chair, wishing so desperately that you were still in it.

I don't know if I'll ever stop wondering—why didn't you call me? Why didn't you reach out? I would have been there in a heartbeat. No questions asked. No judgment. Just us, the way it always was.

But part of me also knows why. Because I've felt it, too.

I know how impossible it felt. I know the weight of the shame, the exhaustion of trying to keep up appearances while addiction slowly suffocates you from the inside. And I especially know how hard it is when you're a therapist. When you're supposed to have the answers. When you spend your days helping others unravel their pain but feel like you have nowhere safe to put your own.

The stigma alone is enough to make you drown in silence. The fear of exposure, of judgment, of condemnation from the powers that be…of losing your license, your career, your identity—it can all be so suffocating. And yet, it can feel like there is nowhere to turn.

Losing you broke my heart in a deeply personal way but what makes it even harder is knowing that this grief extends far beyond just you and I. Your suicide is just one of far too many. Most go unreported, buried beneath quiet obituaries that fail to mention the truth. Mental health professionals are dying, and no one is talking about it.

Therapists. Counselors. Social workers. Psychologists. Behavioral health specialists. We sit with people in their darkest moments. We walk with them through their pain. We hold space for their trauma. We are the anonymous frontliners. Where is our support when we struggle with the disease of substance use disorder?

Physicians have the Physician Health Program.
Lawyers have the Legal Assistance Program.
Pilots have the HIMS program.

Ironic, isn't it? We are the ones who provide the emotional and behavioral support for these professionals, in addition to everyone else. And yet, mental health professionals have no widely established, confidential system of support.

Sure, there are licensing accountability boards, ethics committees, and mandated reporting structures. But where is the space for the therapist who is drowning? Where is the safe, stigma-free, confidential place for a counselor who needs help before they hit rock bottom? Hopefully we have our own therapists—that's essential to do the job—but that doesn't meet the spectrum of intervention needed for substance use disorder.

We can't just walk into an AA meeting or public outpatient program. Not when there's a very real chance we'll run into a client. Not when the very people we're supposed to be helping might suddenly view us as compromised, as broken, as unfit to do our jobs. We would risk being reported to the board, losing our licenses, and losing our ability to do the work we love.

And even if we were willing to take that risk, it wouldn't be ethical. Sitting in a room full of people we are meant to serve, sharing our personal struggles, crossing boundaries that are never supposed to be crossed—that would be a violation of everything we have been trained to uphold.

You and I both know the truth: substance use disorder does not discriminate. It doesn't care how educated you are, how successful you've been, how many people you've helped. It is a biological, neurological, and psychological *disease* that cuts across every ethnicity, socioeconomic status, gender, and profession.

And yet, even within our own field, we pretend like we're somehow supposed to be immune. We're not. If anything, we're more at risk.

You and I spoke countless times about both the blessings and the burdens of this work. How rewarding it is to see people heal, to witness transformation. But also, how exhausting it can be. How devastating it is to feel helpless when we can't reach someone. How sometimes, at the end of the day, it felt like there was nothing left of us to give.

There were so many days we would get together, drink in hand, laughing through our exhaustion and joking about how we were being "sucked dry" by the weight of other people's pain. And in those moments, we would dream about escaping—just running away from it all. Then we'd chuckle and jump to a different topic—steering away from anything that might slip into admitting we were nearing our breaking points.

I know you suffered in silence, like each of us does, under crushing pressure. Burned out, ashamed, and hiding—even from your closest friend. If only you had known…even in your darkest place, you were not alone. Alcoholism just fools us into believing we are. After you left, I learned that a survey done last year found that forty percent of mental health professionals reported feeling burnt out, with seven percent reporting suicidal ideation.

It's no longer a secret that people in our field are at higher risk for suicide. But what remains largely unknown—or at least rarely talked about—is how often substance use disorder is part of that equation. It's the *closet secret* that families and colleagues cover up out of "respect"—or maybe out of denial. It's the part of the story that gets left out of memorials, left out of statistics, left out of the broader conversation.

People don't want to think about the fact that someone as amazing as you is more likely to kill themself than go through the risks and humiliation of trying to get help.

But ignoring it doesn't make it go away.

I wish you could have held on long enough to see the *other side* of all that pain. I wish you could have made it through the fire to experience what I now know to be true. Life on the other side of addiction is more beautiful than one could ever imagine.

I wish I could have held your hand through the fear and shame, through the discomfort of detox, through the crushing vulnerability of surrendering to treatment. I wish I could have helped you see that the thing we fear most—being exposed—is not nearly as terrifying as the illusion we've built around it.

Yes, it was painful. Yes, I felt humiliated at times. But in the end, receiving help was not my downfall—it was my rebirth.

The people who truly loved me did not abandon me—they embraced me. My career did not end. My life did not collapse. In fact, I found a better life—a more authentic, more peaceful, more connected life than I had ever known before.

Sometimes, in my dreams, we get to share this fresh new life together—laughing, exploring, immersed in glorious mysteries. As for my waking life, I will keep your chair here because I never want to forget—any of it. There are no words for how much I miss you. I would give anything to hear your voice again. To laugh with you. To talk with you the way we used to.

But since I can't…I will keep speaking for you. I will keep telling our story. I will do what I can to change things—to stop these tragedies and losses from happening.

We all need to do better. We need support for therapists and mental health professionals. We need better, confidential recovery programs for people in the helping professions. We need to stop treating substance use disorder like a personality weakness or moral failing and start recognizing it as the disease it is. We need to stop pretending we're immune—or that we *should* be.
Because we're not. And too many of us are dying. Recovery is not just possible—it's beautiful. And I would give anything for you to be here to experience it with me.

Instead, I'm sitting in this unbearable silence. With this unbearable loss. Staring at this empty chair that will never be filled again.

I miss you.
I love you.
And I will never stop wishing you had stayed.

Always,

- *L*

A Letter to You: The Path to Recovery and a Better Life

Dear Reader,

If you've made it to this final letter, I want to take a moment to acknowledge you. Whether you're here because you're struggling, because someone you love is, or because you want to understand this disease better, I see you. I know how heavy all of this can feel, and I know the quiet battles that are fought in the shadows—especially for those of us in the helping professions.

If you are struggling with substance use disorder (SUD) and you are a mental health professional, medical professional, first responder, or in any other helping field where anonymity is crucial, I need you to hear this: **You can recover.** You can get your life back. You can heal—not just enough to scrape by, but enough to thrive, to feel whole again. I know because I've lived it.

The Path to Recovery: What You Need to Know

If you are in active addiction and reading this, you likely feel overwhelmed, terrified, or even resigned to your circumstances. I remember those feelings well. I also remember the suffocating fear of exposure—the dread that if I admitted the truth, I would lose everything.

Here's the bigger truth: **Healing is possible, but it requires surrender.** You cannot do this alone. So where do you begin?

1. Seek Treatment—Not Just Any Treatment, But the Right One

You deserve the highest quality of care. Your profession does not disqualify you from receiving real medical treatment for this disease—**it demands that you get it.** Find a **reputable, evidence-based treatment center** that offers:

- **Medication-Assisted Treatment (MAT)** – This is not "swapping one drug for another." Medications like Naltrexone, Gabapentin, or Clonidine can be life-saving tools in your recovery. If opioid use is

185

a factor, alternative options like Suboxone or Methadone may be considered.

- **Research-Based Modalities** – Cognitive Behavioral Therapy (CBT), Motivational Interviewing, trauma-informed care, and other proven interventions will help you understand and change addictive thinking patterns. Finding a center that recognizes and works with the spiritual aspects of our life experience is a strong plus.
- **A Strong Medical and Nutritional Component** – Addiction depletes your body in ways you don't even realize. A center that includes medical supervision and nutritional replenishment will give you a better chance at long-term success.
- **Neurotherapy and Brain Healing** – While this is not yet included in most rehab establishments, I believe it is something that will be in the future. Treatments like neurofeedback and neurostimulation can **repair** damaged brain pathways, helping with impulse control, cravings, and emotional regulation. You are not just treating your behavior—you are healing your brain.

This disease lives in your body, your brain, and your nervous system. Treat all of it.

2. Commit to an Intensive Outpatient Program (IOP)

Rehab is not the finish line—it's the starting block. After inpatient treatment, you need **continued, structured support** in an IOP that includes:

- **Ongoing therapy (individual and group)**
- **Medical and psychiatric support**
- **Accountability in early sobriety**
- **Guidance for navigating work and personal relationships in recovery**

This step is **non-negotiable** for those of us in professions where high-functioning addiction is the norm. You need a bridge from inpatient care to the real world, one that won't let you slip through the cracks.

3. Get Physically and Mentally Healthy

Once you are sober, your **brain and body need time to heal.** Your emotions will be raw, your nervous system dysregulated, and your dopamine system depleted. This is **not a sign of failure—it's biology.**

- **Nutrition and gut health matter** – Your gut is your "second brain" and directly impacts mood, cravings, and mental clarity. Work with a professional who understands nutrition as it relates to addiction recovery.
- **Movement is medicine** – Exercise, yoga, or simply getting outside can strengthen reward pathways in your brain.
- **Neurotherapy and brain stimulation** – If you can access treatments like neurofeedback, neurostimulation, and other verified neurotherapy programs, do it. These therapies help repair the brain and nervous system profoundly impacted by the disease.

4. Report Your SUD to Your Licensing Board—When You Are Ready

This step feels impossible. I won't lie—it's terrifying. But **it's necessary.** Once you are stable in your recovery (which for me was two years after my successful rehab), **you must disclose your substance use disorder to your licensing board** (whether you are a therapist, doctor, nurse, or other licensed professional). I know the boards want earlier reporting, but I also know the process is incredibly triggering. If necessary, it is worth taking a break from your practice to get secure in your sobriety. Then move on to the reporting process which may include:

- **Assessments and psychological evaluations** to determine fitness for practice
- **Monitoring and follow-up expectations** (which can vary depending on your profession and state regulations)

I know this part feels like punishment, but it's not. It's **protection**—for you and the people you serve. If we truly want to end the stigma, we must start with transparency.

5. Find Your People: Meetings, Groups, and Accountability

Anonymity is crucial for us, which makes traditional support groups tricky.

- **AA, NA, or Other 12-Step Fellowships** – While AA has been life-changing for many, **public in-person meetings can be ethically complicated** if your own clients attend them. Fortunately, there are numerous online groups that can be located in other parts of the world.
- **Alternative Groups** – Consider SMART Recovery, Refuge Recovery, or specialized professionals-only groups. Find a space where you can be **honest and supported.**
- **A Sponsor or Mentor** – **You need someone who gets it.** Someone you can call when your mind is screaming for relief. Someone who will hold you accountable but won't judge you.

6. Work the Steps—Or Find Another Structure for Long-Term Growth

Twelve-step programs aren't for everyone, but the **principles behind them are invaluable.** Whether you choose AA, SMART Recovery, or another program, you need **a framework for personal growth.**

- **Do the work** – Recovery isn't just about quitting drinking or using. It's about healing from the inside out.
- **Make amends (when appropriate)** – Carrying shame will eat you alive. A structured way to release it is crucial.
- **Live differently** – Recovery is not just about abstinence. It's about transformation.

You are not alone

I know it feels like you have to do this alone. That's the biggest lie addiction tells us. The reality? There is help. There are resources. There is a way forward.

We are not meant to suffer in silence. You do not have to figure this out by yourself.
If you are reading this and you are struggling, I hope this letter reaches you in time. I hope you make the choice to begin the path of recovery.

I hope you choose life.

With all my love,

- *L*

The Truth About Addiction - Statistics

The #1 Preventable Cause of Death in the U.S.

- Overdoses are now the leading cause of accidental and preventable death—surpassing car accidents, suicides, and gun violence.
- 2023 overdose deaths: 107,000 people (CDC)
- Fentanyl is the leading cause of death for Americans ages 18-49.

The Alcohol Crisis We Don't Talk About

- Alcohol-related deaths have increased 43% since 2006—and they continue to rise.
- 140,000 Americans die every year from alcohol-related causes.
- One person dies every 4 minutes due to alcohol.
- 1 in 3 liver transplants in the U.S. is due to alcohol-related liver disease.

One in Six—Who's Affected?

- 49 million people (or 17.1% of the U.S. population) have a substance use disorder (SUD).
- Nearly 29 million struggle with Alcohol Use Disorder (AUD).
- Over 27 million have a Drug Use Disorder (DUD).
- 7.5 million people suffer from both alcohol and drug addiction.

Addiction Disproportionately Affects Communities of Color

- Overdoses are rising fastest among Black, Latinx, and Native American populations.
- Overdose rates in Black communities grew faster than in white communities between 2018-2020.
- Native Americans experience overdose deaths at rates 27.4% higher than the national average.
- And yet, these communities have less access to treatment.

The System Is Broken

- Fewer than 5% of people who need treatment actually receive it.
- Even fewer receive evidence-based, research-backed care.

- Medication-assisted treatment (MAT) is one of the most effective treatments for addiction, yet...
  - 60% of residential treatment centers don't offer any MAT at all.
  - Only 1% of all facilities offer all three FDA-approved medications for opioid addiction.

Doctors and Insurance Are Failing Patients

- Medical professionals are NOT adequately trained to treat addiction.
  - Only 1 in 4 physicians and nurse practitioners receive any training on addiction in medical school.
  - Even those who do, receive minimal education.
- Insurance is a massive barrier to treatment.
  - Only 60% of employer-sponsored health plans cover addiction treatment at all.
  - Many require prior authorization, delaying access to life-saving care.

What Needs to Change?

✔ We need addiction training for all medical and mental health professionals.
✔ We need insurance to cover comprehensive treatment, just like it would for any other disease.
✔ We need to change the stigma—addiction is not a moral failing, it is a disease.

Final Thoughts:

We don't have time to wait.

Addiction is not just someone else's problem. It is an epidemic.

We need to demand better. We need to make noise. We need to educate, advocate, and take action—before millions more lives are lost.

Resources for Getting Help

Emergency & Crisis Hotlines

These hotlines provide **immediate** crisis support for those struggling with addiction, mental health concerns, or suicidal thoughts.

Suicide & Crisis Support

- **988 Suicide & Crisis Lifeline** – Call or Text **988**
  Website: 988lifeline.org
  Confidential support for anyone in distress, 24/7.
- **Crisis Text Line** – Text **HELLO** to **741741**
  Website: www.crisistextline.org
  24/7 text-based crisis support.
- **Veterans Crisis Line** – Call **988, then Press 1** or Text **838255**
  Website: www.veteranscrisisline.net
  Support for U.S. military veterans and their families.

Substance Use Disorder & Addiction Helplines

- **SAMHSA's National Helpline** – Call **1-800-662-HELP (4357)**
  Website: www.samhsa.gov/find-help/national-helpline
  Free, confidential 24/7 treatment referral and information for individuals and families facing SUD or mental health issues.
- **Partnership to End Addiction – Helpline** – Call **855-378-4373** or Text **CONNECT** to **55753**
  Website: drugfree.org
  Personalized support for families struggling with a loved one's addiction.
- **Shatterproof Addiction Support**
  Website: www.shatterproof.org
  Nationwide advocacy, education, and recovery support resources.

Find a Rehabilitation Treatment Center

These resources help locate **quality treatment centers** that provide evidence-based addiction care.

- **SAMHSA's Treatment Locator**
  Website: www.findtreatment.gov
  Search for nearby addiction treatment facilities, including inpatient, outpatient, and medication-assisted treatment (MAT).
- **Psychology Today's Treatment Directory**
  Website: www.psychologytoday.com/us/treatment-rehab
  Find accredited addiction treatment centers, therapists, and support groups.
- **American Society of Addiction Medicine (ASAM) Treatment Locator**
  Website: www.treatmentatlas.org
  Find evidence-based addiction treatment providers.
- **National Association of Addiction Treatment Providers (NAATP) Directory**
  Website: www.naatp.org
  Trusted rehab centers meeting high ethical standards.

Professional Support for Helping Professions (Confidential Help)

These organizations provide **discreet** recovery support for professionals in high-risk fields.

- **Physician Health Programs (PHPs) – For Medical Professionals**
  Website: www.fsphp.org
  Confidential peer support and addiction treatment referrals for doctors, nurses, and medical personnel.
- **Lawyers Assistance Programs (LAPs) – For Legal Professionals**
  Website: www.americanbar.org/groups/lawyer_assistance
  Confidential help for lawyers, judges, and law students struggling with addiction.
- **International Doctors in AA (IDAA) – Recovery for Healthcare Professionals**
  Website: www.idaa.org
  A fellowship of doctors and healthcare professionals in recovery.
- **Therapist Support Network (For Mental Health Professionals)**
  Website: www.psychotherapynetworker.org
  Education, forums, and support groups for therapists experiencing burnout, addiction, or mental health struggles.

Find a Meeting or Ongoing Recovery Support

Ongoing support is **crucial** for maintaining sobriety. Here are some options:

- **Alcoholics Anonymous (AA) Meeting Finder**
  Website: www.aa.org/find-aa
  Find local or online AA meetings.
- **Narcotics Anonymous (NA) Meeting Finder**
  Website: www.na.org/meetingsearch
  Locate in-person or virtual NA meetings.
- **SMART Recovery (Science-Based Alternative to AA/NA)**
  Website: www.smartrecovery.org
  Non-12-step, evidence-based recovery support groups.
- **Refuge Recovery (Buddhist-Inspired Recovery)**
  Website: www.refugerecovery.org
  Mindfulness and meditation-based recovery program.
- **Celebrate Recovery (Christian-Based Recovery Program)**
  Website: www.celebraterecovery.com
  Faith-based 12-step support groups for addiction and mental health.

Educational Resources for Understanding & Treating SUD

If you want to deepen your knowledge about addiction, treatment, and recovery, check out these resources.

- **National Institute on Drug Abuse (NIDA)**
  Website: www.drugabuse.gov
  Research-based facts about substance use disorders and treatments.
- **SAMHSA (Substance Abuse and Mental Health Services Administration)**
  Website: www.samhsa.gov
  Government agency providing addiction treatment resources, research, and policy updates.
- **American Society of Addiction Medicine (ASAM)**
  Website: www.asam.org
  Educational resources and professional training in addiction medicine.

- **Shatterproof Addiction Treatment Guide**
  Website: www.shatterproof.org/addiction-treatment
  A guide to choosing effective treatment for SUD.
- **Addiction Technology Transfer Center (ATTC) Network**
  Website: www.attcnetwork.org
  Training and research for mental health and addiction professionals.
- **The Recovery Research Institute (Harvard Medical School)**
  Website: www.recoveryanswers.org
  Evidence-based addiction recovery research and education.

You Are Not Alone...

If you or someone you love is struggling with addiction, **help is available.** You are not beyond hope, and you do not have to do this alone. Recovery is possible, and resources exist to guide you every step of the way. **Reach out. Ask for help. Take the first step.**

References

Books & Published Works

- **Alcoholics Anonymous World Services.** (1939). *Alcoholics Anonymous (The Big Book).*
- **American Medical Association (AMA).** (1956, 1987). *Official Classification of Alcoholism and Addiction as Diseases.*
- **Brown, B.** (2010). *The Gifts of Imperfection: Let Go of Who You Think You're Supposed to Be and Embrace Who You Are.* Hazelden Publishing.
- **Brown, B.** (2012). *Daring Greatly: How the Courage to Be Vulnerable Transforms the Way We Live, Love, Parent, and Lead.* Penguin Random House.
- **Einstein, A.** (Various works on science and philosophy). *No problem can be solved from the same level of consciousness that created it.*
- **Frankl, V. E.** (1946). *Man's Search for Meaning.* Beacon Press.
- **Hahn, T. N.** (2017). *The Art of Living.* HarperOne.
- **Hunter, T.** (n.d.). *Anything that is not love is only a visitor to your body.*
- **Ladinsky, D.** (1999). *The Gift: Poems by Hafiz, the Great Sufi Master.* Penguin Compass.
- **Ladinsky, D.** (2011). *A Year with Hafiz: Daily Contemplations.* Penguin.
- **Maté, G.** (2008). *In the Realm of Hungry Ghosts: Close Encounters with Addiction.* North Atlantic Books.
- **Milam, J. R., & Ketcham, K.** (1981). *Under the Influence: A Life-Saving Guide to the Myths and Realities of Alcoholism.* Bantam.
- **O'Donohue, J.** (1999). *Eternal Echoes: Exploring Our Hunger to Belong.* HarperCollins.
- **Palmer, P.** (2018). *On the Brink of Everything: Grace, Gravity, and Getting Old.* Berrett-Koehler Publishers.
- **Ruiz, D. M.** (1997). *The Four Agreements: A Practical Guide to Personal Freedom.* Amber-Allen Publishing.
- **Smith, C., & Hunt, J.** (2021). *Understanding Addiction: Know Science, No Stigma.* Visualize Publishing.
- **White Bison, Inc.** (2006). *The Red Road to Wellbriety.* White Bison, Inc.

Medical & Psychological Research

- **Bresler, D.** (2005). Physiological Consequences of Guided Imagery. *Practical Pain Management, 5*(6).
- **Bogenschutz, M. P., Forcehimes, A. A., Pommy, J. A., Wilcox, C. E., Barbosa, P. C. R., & Strassman, R. J.** (2015). Psilocybin-assisted treatment for alcohol dependence: A proof-of-concept study. *Journal of Psychopharmacology, 29*(3), 289–299. https://doi.org/10.1177/0269881114565144
- **Parodi, K. B., Holt, M. K., Green, J. G., Porche, M. V., Koenig, B., & Xuan, Z.** (2022). Time trends and disparities in anxiety among adolescents, 2012-2018. *Social Psychiatry and Psychiatric Epidemiology, 57*(1), 127-137. https://doi.org/10.1007/s00127-021-02122-9
- **Thomas, K., Malcolm, B., & Lastra, D.** (2017). Psilocybin-Assisted Therapy: A Review of a Novel Treatment for Psychiatric Disorders. *Journal of Psychoactive Drugs, 49*(3), 200-208. https://doi.org/10.1080/02791072.2017.1320734
- **Zhornitsky, S., Oliva, H. N. P., Jayne, L. A., Allsop, A. S. A., Kaye, A. P., Potenza, M. N., & Angarita, G. A.** (2023). Changes in synaptic markers after administration of ketamine or psychedelics: A systematic scoping review. *Frontiers in Psychiatry, 14.* https://doi.org/10.3389/fpsyt.2023.1197890
- **American Psychiatric Association (APA).** (2025). *© 2025 American Psychiatric Association. All Rights Reserved.* 800 Maine Avenue, S.W., Suite 900, Washington, DC 20024. 202-559-3900. apa@psych.org.

- **Lit, R.** (2023, March 13). What Happens When You Meditate. *Stanford Magazine, Stanford University*. https://stanfordmag.org

Religious & Philosophical Texts

- **The Holy Bible** (New International Version). Proverbs 4:23.
- **The Holy Bible** (New International Version). Romans 5:5.
- **Heraclitus of Ephesus.** (6th Century BCE). *Change is the only constant.*

Film & Pop Culture

- **Markus, C., McFeely, S., & Petroni, M.** (2010). *Voyage of the Dawn Treader* (Screenplay adaptation of C.S. Lewis' *The Chronicles of Narnia*).

Statistical & Government Reports

- **Centers for Disease Control and Prevention (CDC).** (2023). *Annual Drug Overdose & Alcohol-Related Death Reports.* www.cdc.gov
- **Shatterproof.org.** *Addiction Statistics & Policy Reform.*
- **New York State Office of Addiction Services and Supports (OASAS).** www.osc.ny.gov
- **Get Smart About Drugs (DEA).** www.getsmartaboutdrugs.gov
- **JAMA Network.** *Medical Research on Addiction and Treatment Accessibility.* www.jamanetwork.com
- **University of Colorado Anschutz Medical Campus (CU Anschutz).** *News & Research on Substance Use Disorders.* news.cuanschutz.edu

Poetry & Miscellaneous Quotes

- **Hunter, T.** *Anything that is not love is only a visitor to your body.*
- **Hafiz.** *Know the true nature of your beloved. In his loving eyes, hear every thought, word, and movement as always, always, beautiful.*

Acknowledgments & Additional Influences

This book has been influenced by a variety of voices in psychology, medicine, spirituality, and literature, with insights drawn from personal experience, academic research, and professional expertise in addiction recovery. Special thanks to my mentors Shahn McGuire, Michael Malone, Bliss Holland and Dr. Yvonne Christman, who brought many of these wonderful teachings to me. I am also grateful to the people and programs at A Way Forward recovery support, who provided numerous educational opportunities and experiences that resulted in some of these valuable insights. I am so very thankful for my family who offered love and support in a multitude of ways, from emotional support and helpful feedback to professional editing and scientific contributions. I am truly blessed to be surrounded by such amazing people!

My gratitude also extends to all the authors, researchers, and organizations dedicated to understanding and addressing substance use disorder with compassion, science, and effective treatment approaches.

www.ingramcontent.com/pod-product-compliance
Lightning Source LLC
Chambersburg PA
CBHW031514120626
46545CB00005B/1878